William Bullein's
Dialogue against the Feuer Pestilence.

Early English Text Society.

Extra Series, No. LII.

1888.

(*Reprinted* 1931.)

A Dialogue
against the Feuer Pestilence.

By WILLIAM BULLEIN.

FROM THE EDITION OF
1578,
COLLATED WITH THE EARLIER EDITIONS OF
1564 AND 1573.

EDITED BY

MARK W. BULLEN AND A. H. BULLEN.

PART I.—THE TEXT.

LONDON:
PUBLISHED FOR THE EARLY ENGLISH TEXT SOCIETY
BY HUMPHREY MILFORD, OXFORD UNIVERSITY PRESS,
AMEN HOUSE, E.C. 4.

1888.
(*Reprinted* 1931.)

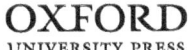
UNIVERSITY PRESS

Great Clarendon Street, Oxford OX2 6DP
United Kingdom

Oxford University Press is a department of the University of Oxford.
It furthers the University's objective of excellence in research, scholarship,
and education by publishing worldwide. Oxford is a registered trade mark of
Oxford University Press in the UK and in certain other countries

© The Early English Text Society 1888

The moral rights of the authors have been asserted

Database right Oxford University Press (maker)

First Edition published in 1888
Reprinted 1931

All rights reserved. No part of this publication may be reproduced,
stored in a retrieval system, or transmitted, in any form or by any means,
without the prior permission in writing of Oxford University Press,
or as expressly permitted by law, or under terms agreed with the appropriate
reprographics rights organization. Enquiries concerning reproduction
outside the scope of the above should be sent to the Rights Department,
Oxford University Press, at the address above

You must not circulate this book in any other form
and you must impose this same condition on any acquirer

Published in the United States of America by Oxford University Press
198 Madison Avenue, New York, NY 10016, United States of America

British Library Cataloguing in Publication Data
Data available

Library of Congress Cataloging in Publication Data
Data available

Extra Series, 52

ISBN 978-0-85-991976-0

NOTE.

The earliest extant edition of William Bullein's *Dialogue* is dated 1564 (8vo.). A unique copy of this edition, which differs considerably from later editions, is preserved in the Britwell Collection; and the editors return their best thanks to Mr. Christie-Miller for his kindness in allowing them to make free use of the precious volume. The *Dialogue*, being full of merry tales (pills to purge melancholy at plague-time), is one of those books that are most easily thumbed out of existence; and it is not surprising that the Britwell copy is unique. On the title-page (which is here reproduced in facsimile) the book is stated to be 'newly corrected'; but occasionally publishers made statements of this kind without any strict regard to truth, in order to push the sale of their ware. Not improbably ed. 1564 is the genuine *editio princeps*. Another edition appeared in 1573,[1] 8vo.; a third in 1578, 8vo.; and the present edition is the fourth.

Nashe in his 'Address to all Christian Readers,' prefixed to *Haue with you to Saffron Walden*, 1596, writes:

"Memorandum, *I frame my whole Booke in the nature of a Dialogue, much like* Bullen *and his Doctor* Tocrub."

This passage shows that the *Dialogue* was well known in 1596; but it must have dropped out of notice shortly afterwards. One might have expected that it would be republished in the plague-year, 1603, when Dekker in *The Wonderfull Yeare* gave his vivid account

---

[1] *A Dialogve bothe pleasaunt and pietifull, wherein is a godlie regiment against the Feuer Pestilence, with a consolation and comforte againste death. Newlie corrected by William Bullein, the authour thereof. Imprinted at London, by Ihon Kingston. Iulij.* 1573.

of the awful visitation; or in 1625, when (as described in Dekker's *A Rod for Runawayes*, and Thomas Brewer's *The Weeping Lady*) London underwent sufferings of exceptional severity. It is to be noticed that Nashe used the edition of 1573 or 1578; for the name "Dr. Tocrub" does not occur in ed. 1564. There can be no doubt that "Dr. Tocrub" was intended (by way of anagram) for Dr. Burcot, an expert in metals and minerals, whose name turns up frequently in the state-papers of the time. It will be remembered that Chettle introduces Dr. Burcot ('though a stranger, yet in England for phisicke famous') in *Kind-Harts Dreame*, n. d. [1593].

The editors are preparing some notes on the *Dialogue*, which, with a biographical and critical memoir of William Bullein, and copious extracts from his remaining works, will form a separate Part.

In the present edition the text of ed. 1578 (from a copy belonging to Mr. Mark W. Bullen) has been followed in the main; and the readings of eds. 1564, 1573 are recorded at the foot of the page. When the previous editions give an obviously better reading, it has been used, and the reading of ed. 1578 noted. It has not been thought advisable to reproduce in modern type the few contractions used by the old printer, their meaning not admitting of doubt in any case. In the labour of collation the editors have been greatly assisted by Mr. W. H. Utley.

Facsimiles of the title-pages of eds. 1564, 1578, are given on the opposite page.

To the right worshipfull

and his singuler frende[1] *Maister*
Edward Barrette of Bel-
hous of Essex, Esquier, Willyam Bulleyn sendeth
salutations.

Right worshipfull Sir, if my[2] Chamber, Hall, Gallerie, or any newe decked house were apparelled or hanged al in one mournyng darcke colour, it would rather moue sorowe then gladnes: but no pleasure to the beholders of the same. Therefore the diuersitie or varietie of pleasaunte colours dooe grace and beautifie the same through the settyng forth of sondrie shapes: and as it were to compell the commers in to beholde the whole worke. Euen so I dooe commende vnto you this little Booke (wherein I writte part thereof in your owne house) which dooe intreate of sonderie thynges to you I dooe hope not vnprofitable, wherein I have shortly described our poore nedie brothers[3] pouertie. Callyng vpon the mercilesse riche, whose whole trust is in the vain riches of this worlde, entangeled as it were emong briers, so that in the hour of death God is farthest from his mynde, and the gooddes euill gotten are worse spent and come to nothyng, at what tyme Phisicke[4] can not preuaile. I haue also not forgotten the shamfull syn which raigneth in this worlde called ingratitude, which linially came from the loines of that false vilain Judas, neither the sicopantes,[5] gnatoes, liars and flatterers of this worlde, the verie poison of the soule. Oh better, saieth Salomon, is

---

[1] Ed. 1564, singulare good frende; ed. 1573, singuler good friende.
[2] Ed. 1564, any.   [3] Eds. 1564, 1573, brother his.
[4] Ed. 1564, no Physicke can; ed. 1573, Phisicke no can.
[5] Eds. 1564, 1573, Sicophantes.

the woundes of the frend then the kisses of the flatterer. Further, how many meanes maie be vsed againste the Pestilence, as good aire, diete, medicines accordingly : the which, if it do not preuaile, then cometh on the merciles power of death ouer all flesh : fearyng no kyng, queene, lorde, ladie, bond, or slaue, but rather maketh all creatures alike to him. Then doe I conclude with the diuine, gods cheef and moste best instrument in the church, &c. And as I do well consider a gentleman of your good Nature can but take youre freendes simple token in good parte, Even so I am sorie that it is no better to plasure you, yet giuyng God moste humble thankes for the same, who keep you in good health & worship.

This twelfe of Marche 1564.

Yours euer, W. Bullein.[1]

Nullus vnquam hominem mortalem beatum indicet antequam bene defunctum viderit.

[1] Eds. 1564 and 1573, William Bulleyn

To the Reader.

Good reader, when aduersitie draweth neare to any Citie or Towne, and the vengeaunce of God appereth either by Hunger, Sicknesse, or the Sworde, then mannes nature is moste fearefull, but yet worldlie prouidence to helpe theimselues: which in the tyme of prosperitie or quietnesse is carelesse and forgetfull, neither myndefull to feare God, nor pitifull[1] to helpe their neighbor in aduersitie. And when thei are touched by the fearfull stroke of the Pestilence of their nexte neighbour, or els in their owne familie, then thei vse Medicines, flie the Aire, &c. Which indeede are verie good meanes, and not against Gods woorde so to doe; then other some falleth into sodaine deuotion, in giuyng almose to the poore and needie, whiche before haue doen nothing els but oppressed theim and haue dooen them wrong: other doe locke[2] from their hartes Gods liuely worde, and refuse grace offered by Christes spirite, thinkyng there is no God. Some other are preuented by death in their flourishyng yeres, which in the crosse of death haue their onely consolation in Jesus Christe. All this is descri-

    bed here in this plain Dia-
    logue: praiyng you pa-
    ciently to take it in
    good parte.
    From
    hym that is yours
    to commaunde,
    W. Bullein.[3]

---

[1] Ed. 1573, pietifull.   [2] Ed. 1564, looke.   [3] Ed. 1564, Bulleyn.

A DIALOGVE.

The Interlocutours are twelue persones.

| { | Mendicus
Ciuis
Vxor
Medicus
Antonius
Roger | } 4 | { | Crispinus
Auarus
Ambodexter
Mendax
Mors
Theologus | } 8 |

Mendicus.

God saue my gud Maister and Maistresse, the Barnes, and all this halie houshaude, and shilde you from all doolle and shem, and sende you comfort of all thynges that you waude haue gud of, and God and our dere Leddie shilde and defende you from this Pest. Our father whiche art in heauen, hallowed be your name;[1] your kyngdome come, your willes[2] bee dooen[3] in yearth as it is in heauen, &c.

Ciuis.

Me thinke I doe heare a good manerly Begger at the doore, and well brought vp. How reuerently he saieth his Pater noster! he thous not God, but you hym. Gods blessyng on his harte! I praie you, wife, giue the poore man somethyng to his dinner.

Vxor.

Sir, I will heare hym saie the Lordes praier better before I giue hym any thing.

Ciuis.

What a reconyng is this! Dame, doe as I commaunde you; he is poore; we haue plentie; he is verie poore and hongrie; therefore dispatche hym a gods name, and let him go.[4]

---

[1] Ed. 1573, names.   [2] Ed. 1564, will.   [3] Ed. 1573, your willes doen.
[4] The words "and let him go" are not in ed. 1564.

Vxor.

Softe fire maketh swete Malte : he shall tary my leasure.

Mendicus.

Maistresse, if you be angrie with the saiyng of my *Patar noster* in Englishe, I will saie it in Latine, and also my *Debrafundis*.[1] But so God helpe me, I do not ken nene of them bethe what thei meane.[2]

Vxor.

I thinke the same : suche Carpenter, suche chips : your Curate is some honest man, I warrant you, and taketh muche pain in feedyng his flock, as semeth by your learning. I praie you, what countrie man be you?

Mendicus.

Sauyng you honour, gud Maistresse, I was borne in Redesdale in Northumberland, and came of a wight ridyng sirname called the Robsons, gud honast men & true, sauyng a little shiftyng for their liuing. God and our Leddie helpe them, silie pure men!

Vxor.

What doest thou here in this[3] Countrie? me thinke thou art a Scot by thy tongue.

Mendicus.

Trowe me neuer mare then, gud deam. I had better bee hangad in a withie or[4] in a cowtaile, then be a rowfooted Scot, for thei are euer fare and fase : I haue been a fellon sharpe manne on my handes in my yonge daies, and brought many of the Scottes to grounde in the Northe Marches, and gaue them many greisly woundes; ne manne for manne durste abide my[5] luke, I was so fell. Then the limmer Scottes hared me, burnt my guddes, and made deadlie feede on[6] me and my barnes, that now I haue nethyng but this sarie bagge and this staffe, and the charitie of sike gud people as you are, gud Maistresse : Ause I haue many of my sirename here in the Citie that wade thinke ne shem on me, yea, honast handcraftie men.

---

[1] Ed. 1564, Deprofundis; ed. 1573, De brafundis.
[2] "what thei meane"—not in ed. 1564.
[3] So ed. 1564.—Ed. 1573, thie; ed. 1578, the. [4] Ed. 1564, of a cowtaile.
[5] Eds. 1564, 1573, me. [6] Ed. 1564, with.

Ciuis.

How gotte you in at the gates, my good freende?

Mendicus.

Deare sir, I haue many Cuntrith men in this faire Citie that came of honest stock in our lande, and some beyonde[1] vs twentie or thirtie lange[2] miles, that make[3] pure shift in the citie and in the countrie ause. I came in ne place, but either the Parsone, Bailie, Conestable, or cheef of the Parishe is of our cuntrith borne, and same[4] pure men as mine awne self, God ken. Emong whom the Bedle of the Beggers beyng a Ridesdale man borne, a gud man and a true, which for ill will in his youth did fleem[5] the Countrie, it was laied to his charge the driuyng of kine hem to his Fathers byre. But Christe knaweth he was sackless, and liue as honestly in his age as his sire did when he was yong, gud maister.

Ciuis.

I was borne in the North, my felowe, and doe liue here in this Citie. I came hether when I was yonge, and when I was verie poore, but now I am in good case to liue emong the reste of my neighbours. I[6] thank God for it.

Mendicus.

Gods benison on you, and our deare Leddies. I came[7] hether purely in myne age; I haue nethyng but wedom, we ladie,[8] weesme.[9]

Vxor.

Giue God onely thankes, for so is his holie will and commaundements that we should call vppon hym in the daies of trouble and onely honour hym. We haue no commaundment to honor our Ladie but[10] Christ onely.

Mendicus.

I thinke one waman wade take an other womans parte: doe as it shall please you; I am ne clerke, but an Ingram man of small cideration in suche arogant buke farles.

---

[1] Ed. 1564, a little beyonde.   [2] Omitted in ed. 1564.
[3] Ed. 1564, can make.   [4] Eds. 1564, 1573, some.   [5] Ed. 1564, fleen.
[6] "I thank God for it"—omitted in ed. 1564.   [7] Ed. 1564, come.
[8] Ed. 1573, weladie.   [9] "we ladie, weesme"—omitted in ed. 1564.
[10] "but Christ onely"—omitted in ed. 1564.

Ciuis.

What newes[1] as you come by the waie, Countrie man?

Mendicus.

Nene but aude maners, faire saiynges, fause hartes, and ne deuotion, God amende the market! Miccle tule[2] for the purse, decieuyng of eche other. In the countrie strife, debate, runnyng for euery trifle to the Lawiers, hauyng nethyng but the nutshelles, the Lawiers eate the carnelles. Ause muche reisyng of rentes and gressomyng of men,[3] causyng greate dearth, muche[4] pouertie. God helpe, God helpe, the warlde is sare chaunged; extortioners, couetous men, and hypocrites doe much[5] preuaile. God cutte them shorter, for thei doe make a blacke warlde, euen hell vpon yearth. I thinke the greate feende or his deam will wearie them all. Nene other newes I ken, but that I did se mucle prouidence made in the countrie for you in the Citie, which doe feare the Pestilence. I met with wagones, Cartes, & Horses full loden[6] with yong barnes, for fear of the blacke Pestilence, with their boxes of Medicens and sweete perfumes. O God, how fast did thei run by hundredes, and were afraied of eche other for feare of smityng.

Ciuis.

I haue some of my children forthe, God sende them well to speede.

Mendicus.

Maister, why goe you not with theim your self?

Ciuis.

No, youth are apte to take the Plague. And, further, parentes are more naturall to their children then children to their fathers and mothers. Nature dooeth descende, but not ascende. Also if the citezen should depart when[7] the Plague dooe come, then there should not onely be no Plague in the Citie, but also the Citie should be voide and emptie for lacke of the inhabitauntes[8] therein, therefore Goddes will bee doen emong his people. I doe not intende[9] to flee;

---

[1] Ed. 1564, in the Countree as, &c. [2] Ed. 1564, moche toilyng.
[3] Ed. 1564, "and gressomyng of men" omitted. [4],[5] Ed. 1564, mucle.
[6] So ed. 1573.—Ed. 1564, ladē; ed. 1578, londen.
[7] Eds. 1564, 1573, when as. [8] Eds. 1564, 1573, inhabitours.
[9] Ed. 1578, incende.

notwithstandyng, I praie God of his mercie deliuer vs from this
Plague, for if it doe continewe, God knoweth it will not onely take
awaie a number of poore people, but many wealthie and lustie
Marchauntes also.

Mendicus.

If such plague doe ensue it is no greate losse. For, firste, it shall
not onely deliuer the miserable poore man, woman, and barnes[1] from
hurte and carefulnesse into a better warlde, but ause cutte of many
coueteous vsurers, whiche bee like fat vncleane swine, whiche
dooe neuer good vntill thei come to the dishe, but wroote out
euery plante that thei can come by; and like vnto greate stinkyng
mucle medin hilles, whiche neuer doe pleasure vnto the Lande or
grounde vntill their heapes are caste abroade to the profites of
many, whiche are kepte neither to their owne comfortes nor others,
but onely[2] in beheading[3] them; like vnto cruell Dogges liyng in a
Maunger, neither eatyng the Haye theim selues ne sufferyng the
Horse to feed thereof hymself. And in sike plagues we pure people
haue muccle[4] gud. Their losse is our lucke[5]; when thei dooe become
naked, we then are clethed againste their willes; with their dooles
and almose we are reliued; their sickness is our health, their death[6]
our life. Besides vs pakers,[7] many me men haue gud lucke, as the
Vicre,[8] Parishe Clarke, and the Belle man; often tymes the Executours bee no losers by this game. And in fine, in my fantasie it is
happy to the Huntman when he haue nethyng of the Catte but the
sillie skinne. We beggers recke[9] nought of the carcas of the dead
body, but doe defie it; we looke for aude caste coates, Jackettes,[10]
Hose, Cappes, Beltes, and Shoes by their deathes, which in their
liues thei waude not departe from, and this is our happe. God[11] sende
me of them.

Ciuis.

Goe thy waies to *Antonius*[12] gates, For thether euen within this
twoo howers I did see maister *Tocrub*[13] solempnely ridyng vpon his

---

[1] Ed. 1564, barne.   [2] Ed. 1564, enely.   [3] Eds. 1564, 1573, behadyng.
[4] Ed. 1564, micke.   [5] Ed. 1564, gaine.
[6] So ed. 1564.—Eds. 1573, 1578, dede.   [7] Ed. 1564, beggers.
[8] Ed. 1564, Curate.   [9] Ed. 1564, couet nought for.
[10] Ed. 1564, dublettes.   [11] "God sende," &c.—omitted in ed. 1594.
[12] Ed. 1564, Antonius Mantuanus.   [13] Ed. 1564, Antonius Capistranus.

mule, with a side goune, a greate chaine of gold about his necke, his Apothicarie *Crispine*,[1] a neighboures childe borne hereby in Barbarie,[2] and his little Lackey, a proper yong applesquire called *Pandarus*, whiche carrieth the keye of his[3] Chamber with hym. These are all gone in at the gates to that noble Italian. His stewarde[4] this daie, because his maister is[5] verie sicke, applied the poore menne with the purse with muche deuotion for the tyme, beyng without hope of his maisters recouery.

Mendicus.

I praie God sende vs many sike praies, for it is merie with vs when ene[6] mannes hurte doe turne to many mennes gaines. I will go thether; fare you well, gud maister. I will drawe nere, and herken what mayster doctor will say, if I might be in place.

Ciuis.

Farewell, for thou doest not care which ende doe goe forwarde so that thy tourne may be serued.

Medicus.

How dooe you, good Maister *Antonius*? Lorde God, howe are you chaunged! How chaunceth this? What is the matter that you looke so pale? You did send for mee by your seruaunte *Iohannes*,[7] a gentle young man, which lamenteth[8] muche for you; when[9] I heard it, with all speede I came from my other pacients, of whom I thinke I haue taken myne *vltimum vale*.

Antonius.

You are welcome, Maister doctour, with all my harte; now helpe at a pinche, or els neuer, for I doe feare my selfe verie much. Oh, my harte!

Medicus.

I warraunt you, man, let mee feele your pulse, and then shall I procede to the cure with medicine and diet accordingly.

Antonius.

Take your pleasure, good Maister Doctour; here is my hande,

---

[1] Ed. 1564, Senior Crispinus; ed. 1573, Crispinus.
[2] Barbican?   [3] Ed. 1564, the.   [4] Ed. 1564, aulmner.   [5] Ed. 1564, was.
[6] Ed. 1578, eny.   [7] Ed. 1564, Iohannes de Corsica.
[8] Ed. 1564, lamented.   [9] Eds. 1564, 1573, and when.

feele my pulse, and then you shall see myne Vrine, and knowe the tyme of my sickness.

Medicus.

These are no verie good tokens, neither in your Vrine, Pulse, Stoole, &c. But I wil doe the best for you that I can doe by arte.

Antonius.

And then you shall wante no golde, for though I lacke health,[1] yet I want no golde of euery coigne, and siluer also. My warehouses are well fitted[2] with wares of sondrie kindes, which I doe sell vnto the retailers. Further, I haue wares of most aunciciet seruice, whiche owe me nothyng, bothe in packes, vesselles, and chestes, &c., which are not fitte for the retailers. Them do I kepe for shiftes when any gentlemen or longe suter in the Lawe are behinde hand, and knowe not what to doe: then by good sureties, or assured landes by Statute Marchaunt, &c., I doe sometyme make thirtie or fourtie[3] in the hundred by yere. I haue diuerse suche honeste wayes to liue vppon, through the wittie and secrete handelyng of my Brokers here in the Citee, and my Factours which are at Antwarpe, &c., By whom I do vnderstande the state, and what commoditie is beste. Further, I haue extended vpon aunciente landes in the Countrie for the breach of couenauntes, That, to conclude with you, maister Doctor, I could neuer haue died in a worse tyme, my busines is such. I would of all thinges liue still, for here I do knowe what I haue and how I am vsed, but when I am gone I doe not knowe what shall happen vnto me, nor whom to trust with that[4] which I haue gotten with trauell and obtained by fortune.

Medicus.

You doe speake like a wise man as euer I heard, and moste thynges that you haue taken in hand haue greate profite with you. Of my parte, I would bee lothe to lose you, bothe for an vnfained loue that I doe beare vnto you for your wisedome, and also for your liberalitie and giftes giuen to me many a time. Lo, here is the Damaske goune yet in store. Here is also a Flagone chaine of the hundred angelles that you did giue me in your laste greate Feuer.

---

[1] Ed. 1564, helpe; ed. 1578, heath. [2] Eds. 1564, 1573, filled.
[3] Ed. 1564, XXX or L. [4] Ed. 1564, y^t.

Antonius.

Who is able to resist suche a multitude of angells? I thinke fewe doctours of Phisicke. But rather then I would dye I wil let flie a thousande more, for these are the Angelles that shall keepe mee.[1]

Medicus.

That is the waie, I assure you, to perfite health; for[2] that cause the Phisician was ordeined, as it is written: Honour the Phisician with the honor that is due vnto hym because of necessitie, for the lord hath[3] created hym; and hee shall receiue giftes of the kyng, yea, and of all men.[4]

Antonius.

That is a good swete text for Phisicians; but why doe you leaue out these wordes in the middes of the matter, which is, Of the most highest commeth learnyng? And so I doe remember I heard our Curate reade in the Churche, as by chaunce I came in with a Sergeant to arest a debter of mine.[5]

Medicus.

What your Curate pleased hym to read I care not, for I meddle with no Scripture matter[6] but to serue my tourne. But[7] that whiche I haue saied is written in the Bible, I haue heard saie so.[8]

Antonius.

Be all thinges written in the Bible true? I praie you tell mee.

Medicus.

God forbidde, Maister Antonius! then it would make a fraie emong Marchauntes; for it is written,[9] None shall enter into gods dwellyng, or rest with hym vppon his holie[10] mountaine, that lendeth his money vpon vsurie, or to vsurie whereby to hinder his neighbour. And this is nowe become the greatest trade, And many be vndoen by borowyng, and fewe doe lose by lendyng, specially men of your worshipfull experience. And how like you this texte?

[1] The words "for these are the Angelles," &c., are not in ed. 1564.
[2] Eds. 1564, 1573, and for.   [3] Ed. 1564, haue.
[4] The words "yea, and of all men" are not in ed. 1564.
[5] Ed. 1564, twoo Bankeroutes.   [6] Eds. 1564, 1573, matters.
[7] Ed. 1564, But *I knowe* that which, &c.
[8] The words "I haue heard saie so" do not occur in ed. 1564.
[9] In the margin of ed. 1564 is "Psal. xv."; in the margin of ed. 1573, "Psalm 23."   [10] "holie" omitted in ed. 1564.

Antonius.

Texte how they will texte, I will trust none of them all, say what they will; there be many such sayings against men, as the ten Commandementes, &c. Well, for my part I haue little to doe in these matters; mary, I would be glad to liue orderly and ciuillie, so that the worlde should not wonder at my doinges; but if damnation should arise when the scripture doth threaten it to men, then should wittie wordes in bargainyng, with facing othes,[1] and pleasaunt Venerous Table talke, and[2] reuilyng of our enemies, &c., be accompted dampnation. Then I warraunte you helle is well furnished with Courtiers, Marchauntes, Soldiours, Housbandmen, and some of the Cleargie, I warraunt you also, among whom there are many more spitful then spirituall. Euen so[3] there are emong the Phisicians many more coueteous then kind harted. I meane not you, maister doctour Tocrub.[4]

Medicus.

Sir, I doe knowe you doe not; but so God helpe mee, one thing doeth muche rejoyce my harte in your communication.

Antonius.

What is that?

Medicus.

I thinke that we twoo are of one religion.

Antonius.

What is that, I praie you, for I knowe not myne owne religion?

Medicus.

Commaunde your folkes to departe out of the chamber, and your yonge frie[5] also, whiche you haue gotten by chaunce medley, for want of Mariage; for the old Prouerb is, Small Pitchers haue wide eares. And the fielde haue eyes and the woodde eares also.[6] Therefore we must comen closelie, and beware of blabbes. There[7] are many Protestantes.

[1] Ed. 1573 reads "with braggyng." [2] Ed. 1564, with.
[3] Eds. 1564, 1573, euen as. [4] Ed. 1564 reads simply "Maister doctour."
[5] Ed. 1564, scapes. [6] Ed. 1564 reads "& the wood haue eares."
[7] The words "There are," &c., are omitted in ed. 1564.

A DIALOGVE.

Antonius.

Well, now the doores are sparred, say on your mynde. Of what Religion are you? Be plaine with me, man.

Medicus.

Herke in your eare.[1] I am neither Catholike, Papist, nor Protestant,[2] I assure you.

Antonius.

What then? You haue rehearsed choyse and plentie of religions. What do you honour, the Sonne, the Moone, or the Starres? beaste, stone, or foule? fishe or tree?

Medicus.

No, forsothe, I doe none of theim all. To be plain, I am a *Nulla fidian*, and there are many of our secte. Marke our doynges.[3]

Antonius.

Oh, *Qui dixit*[4] *in corde suo non est deus.*[5] Well, we differ verie little in this poincte, but if I doe liue, we shall drawe nere to an vnitie. In the meane tyme, let your Pothecarie prouide some good thinges for the bodie. I praie you open the doore.

Medicus.

Maisters, I pray you call *Crispinus* hether into the galarie, and *Leonardus*[6] with hym.

Crispine.

What is your pleasure, maister Doctour?

Medicus.

How doe you like the[7] gardein?

Crispine.

There are plentie of goodly herbes, both clensing, healyng, losyng, bindyng, and restoryng. I neur did see more choise of sondri kindes of straunge flowers, most pleasaunt to the eye, and sweete also. The fine knottes are doen in[8] good arte, Geometrically figured. A sweete conduit in the middest, made of fine stone, plentifully castyng forthe

---

[1] Ed. 1564, "Herke in your eare, sir."
[2] Ed. 1564, Catholike, Papiste, Protestante nor Auabaptiste.
[3] "marke," &c.—omitted in ed. 1564.   [4] Ed. 1573, dixi.
[5] Ed. 1573 has in margin "Psalm 14."   [6] Ed. 1564, Leonardus de Montano.
[7] Ed. 1564, this.   [8] Ed. 1573, by.

water like fine siluer streames many waies; in which conduite I did beholde by the space of one hower a maruelous thing, the meanyng thereof[1] I knowe not.

Medicus.

What is[2] it, Crispine?

Crispine.

The piller was eight foote square, and xviij foote high, with compartementes of cunnyng masonrie curiously couered with fine golde. Upon the toppe a Tyger fearfully, hauyng a yonge childe in his armes readie to kill it; the childe had a croune of golde upon his head, and in his left hande a globe figuering the whole worlde, and was called μικρόκοσμος,[3] about which was written *Globus conuersus est.*

Medicus.

This gentleman came of a greate house, this is the crest of his armes; for he descended of the most auncient Romains, I warrant you; he is no vpstart, assure your self.

Crispine.

I had thought it had rather signified the conditions of a cruell tyraunt or some bloodie conquerour, whiche by vsurpation getting thy victorie of any common wealth, as landes, countries, or citees, eftsones do spoile the true heires and owners of the lande whiche doe weare the croune, chaunge the state of the Commons to the worser part, spoylyng theim with the[4] sworde and bondage, which appered by these wordes, *Globus conuersus est:* the worlde is chaunged or tourned in suche a common weale.[5]

Medicus.

A good obseruation. What did you see then?

Crispine.

I did beholde on the other[6] side the nine Muses, with strange instrumentes of Musicke, sittyng vnder the hille Parnasus; and Poetes[7] sittyng under the grene trees with Laurell garlandes besette with Roses about their heades, hauyng golden Pennes in their handes, as *Homer, Hesiodus, Ennius,* &c., writyng Verses of sondrie

---

[1] Ed. 1573, whereof. [2] Ed. 1564, was. [3] Ed. 1564, *Microcosmos.*
[4] Ed. 1564, "the" omitted. [5] Ed. 1564, "in suche," &c. omitted.
[6] Ed. 1564, on the one side. [7] Ed. 1564, the poetes.

kindes. And *Lucanus,* sat there very high, nere vnto the cloudes, apparelled in purple, saiyng,

> quantum semotus[1] Eoo[2]
> Cardine, Pernasus gemino petit æthera colle,
> Mons[3] Phœbo Bromioque sacer.

And nere theim satte old Morall Goore with pleasaunt penne in hande, commendyng honest loue without luste, and pleasure without pride; Holinesse in the Cleargie without Hypocrisie,[4] no tyrannie in rulers, no falshode in Lawiers, no Vsurie in Marchauntes, no rebellion in the Commons, and vnitie emong kyngdomes, &c. Skelton satte in the corner of a Piller with a Frostie bitten face, frownyng, and is scante yet cleane cooled of the hotte burnyng Cholour kindeled againste the cankered Cardinall Wolsey; wrytyng many[5] sharpe *Distichons* with bloudie penne againste hym, and sente them by the infernal riuers *Styx, Flegiton,* and *Acheron* by the Feriman of helle, called *Charon,* to the saied Cardinall.

> *How the Cardinall came of nought,*
> *And his Prelacie solde and bought;*
> *And where suche Prelates bee*
> *Sprong of lowe degree,*
> *And spirituall dignitee,*
> *Farewell benignitee,*
> *Farewell simplicitee,*[6]
> *Farewell good charitee!*
> *Thus paruum literatus*
> *Came from Rome gatus,*
> *Doctour dowpatus,*
> *Scante a Bachelaratus:*
> *And thus Skelton did ende*
> *With Wolsey his frende.*

Wittie Chaucer satte in a chaire of gold couered with Roses, writyng Prose and Risme, accompanied with the Spirites of many kynges, knightes, and faire Ladies, whom hee plesauntly besprinkeled with the sweete water of the welle consecrated vnto the Muses, ecleped *Aganippe.* And as the[7] heauenly spirite commended his

---

[1] Old eds., sermotus.   [2] Old eds., ego.
[3] Old eds., Motis. (The quotation is from Book V. of Lucan's *Pharsalia,* ll. 71-3.)   [4] Ed. 1564, "without hypocrisie" omitted.
[5] Eds. 1564, 1573, many a.   [6] Eds. 1564, 1573, have an extra line, "*Farewell, humanitee,*"   [7] Ed. 1564, his.

deare Brigham for the worthy entombing of his bones, worthy of memorie, in the long sleepyng chamber of most famous kinges, Euen so in tragedie he bewailed the sodaine resurrection of many a noble man before their time, in spoyling of Epitaphes, whereby many haue loste their inheritaunce, &c. And further thus he saied lamentyng :—

> *Couetos men do catch al that thei may haue,*
> *The feeld & the flock, the tombe & the graue,*
> *And as they abuse riches, and their graues that are gone,*
> *The same measure they shall haue euery one.*
> *Yet no burial hurteth holy men though beastes them deuour,*
> *Nor riche graue preuaileth the wicked for all yeartlhy power.*

Lamenting Lidgate lurking emong the Lilie[1] with a balde skons, with a garland of Willowes about his pate : booted he was after sainct Benets guise, and a black stamell robe with a lothly monsterous hoode hanging backwarde; his stoopyng forward bewayling euery cstate, with the spirite of prouidence foreseyng the falles of wicked men, and the slipprie seates of princes, the ebbyng and flowyng, the risyng and falling of men in auctoritie, and how vertue doth aduaunce the simple, and vice ouerthrowe the most noble of the worlde. And thus he said :—

> *Oh, noble Princes, conceiue and doe lere*
> *The fall of kynges for misgouernire,*
> *And prudently peisyng of*[2] *this matter,*
> *Virtue is stronger then either plate or maile :*
> *Therefore consider when wisdom doth*[3] *counsaile,*
> *Chief preseruative of Princely magnificence,*
> *Is to Almightie God to doe due reuerence.*

Then Bartlet[4] with an hoopyng Russet, long coate, with a prety hoode in his necke, fine[5] knottes vppon his girdle after Frances trickes. He was borne beyond the colde riuer of Twede. He lodged vppon a sweete bed of Camomill, under the Sinamum tree. Aboute hym many Shepherdes and Sheepe with pleasaunt Pipes; greatly abhorryng the life of Courtiers, Citizens, Usurers, and Banckruptes, &c., whose olde daies are miserable. And the estate of Shepheardes and countrey people he accoumpted most happie and sure, &c., Saiyng :—

[1] Ed. 1564, Lilies. [2] Omitted in eds. 1564, 1573. [3] Eds. 1564, 1573, dooe.
[4] Ed. 1564, Bartley. [5] Ed. 1564, and fiue ; ed. 1573, and fine.

> *Who entreth the court in yong & tender age,*
> *Are lightly blinded with foly and outrage,*
> *But suche as enter with witte and grauitie*
> 4 *Bow not so sone to such enormitie;*
> *But ere*[1] *thei enter, if thei haue lerned nought,*
> *Afterwardes*[2] *Vertue the least of theyr thought.*

[Nexte[3] theim in a blacke chaire of Gette stone, in a coat of 8 armes, sate an aunciente knight in Orange Tawnie as one forsaken, bearyng upon his breast a white Lion, with a Croune of riche golde on his hedde. His name was sir Dauie Linse vppon the mounte, with a hammer of strong steele in his hande, breakyng a 12 sonder the counterfeicte crosse kaies of Rome, forged by Antichriste. And thus this good knight of Scotlande saied to England the elder brother and Scotlande the younger:—

> *Habitare fratres in unum*
> 16 *Is a blesfull thyng,*
> *One God, one faith, one baptisme pure,*
> *One lawe, one lande, and one kyng.*
> *Clappe handes together, brethren dere,*
> 20 *Unfained truce together make,*
> *And like frendes dooe ever acorde,*
> *But French and Romaine doe first forsake.*
> *You are without the continent,*
> 24 *A sole lande of aunciente fame,*
> *Ab origine a people olde,*
> *Bolde Britaines ecleped by name.*
> *Sicut erat in principio.*
> 28 *Graunt, oh God, it maie bee*
> *In saecula saeculorum,*
> *That we maie have peace in thee.*
> *Then we shall feare no forein power*
> 32 *That againste vs shall advaunce,*
> *The Tartre cruell, the curse of Rome,*
> *Ne yet the power of Fraunce, &c.*

On the second square] There[4] was a faire Diall for this Orison, 36 vnto whiche was added the howers of the Planettes: vpon the same was written in large letters of fine gold, *tempora labuntur*.

Medicus.

There stop and lay a strawe; For *Tempora labuntur* is to say,

---

[1] Ed. 1564, or.   [2] Ed. 1564, afterward is.
[3] The whole of the bracketed passage was omitted in eds. 1573, 1578.
[4] Omitted in ed. 1564.

by little and little tyme doth[1] slip awaie. I will heare the reste of the matter at leasure. What is it a clocke?

Crispine.
But early day, scant eight of the clocke.

Medicus.
Well, I praie you dispence all thynges in order, *Contra Pestem*, in the same sorte as you did[2] yesterday, which was giuen to Paule.

Crispine.
Sir, I haue spente all my fine Myrrhe; what shall I doe?

Medicus.
You are a wise man: put in *quid pro quo*, called ἀντιβαλλόμενα. *Hoc est simplicia que aliorum facultati similium penuria subponi possunt medici consilio. Intelligis?*

Crispine.
Etiam, domine doctor.

Medicus.
Moue te ocius et quicquid agas prudenter ages[3] *tu carnifex.*

Crispine.
By God he shall paie for the Malte grindyng; he hath[4] enough, he knoweth no[5] ende of his pelfe. It will come to an euill ende; God sende me more suche cheates. What! me thinke I see twoo men in long gounes with short beardes at the gates. What are they, a Gods name?

Medicus.
I knowe theim verie well; they are two Pettifoggers in the Lawe; the one is called Maister *Auarus*, a good Gentleman and of a greate house, a man of good conscience, in deede he is my cousin germaine on my mothers side: surely hee can giue good counsaile, and is fitte to be with such a man as Maister *Antonius* is: in deede they haue been long acquainted, and will neuer giue ouer vnto the ende. The[6] Rauen will seeke the carrion.

[1] Eds. 1564, 1573, dooe.
[2] Ed. 1564, in the same sort, bothe noumber of the Simples, Dose and quantitee, euen as you did it.
[3] Ed. 1564 reads "agas," for "ages," and omits "tu carnifex."
[4] Ed. 1564, haue.   [5] Ed. 1564, know none.
[6] "The Rauen," &c., omitted in ed. 1564.

Crispine.

Who is the other on the lefte hande? Hee seemeth to bee a proper gentleman and a studious; he is leane, an handsome, clenlie, pretie[1] man. Me thinke he hath[2] on eche side of his goune a Bagge, and his handes[3] in them; he[4] hath also a gogle eye.

Medicus.

Every man hath his grace and gesture. I promise you I durst commit a greate secrete vnto him. Oh, he is a peragon.

Crispine.

What meaneth hee by winkyng like a Goose in the raine, and byting of his lippe?

Medicus.

Doe you note that? it is a good signe of a constant man: marke it when you will, he is a wittie felowe, and one that is in greate estimation, fitte for Master *Antonius;* his name is *Ambodexter.* Goe doune with spede, and saye you haue giuen Maister *Antonius* his Purgation, and this day hee hath[6] no leasure to speake with any man, and also how that he is amended. For if the Curate were here for the soule, wee for the bodie, and *Auarus* for the purse, here were but a madde companie; wee should neuer agree together, but fall into discordes. Dispatch them with speede. fare ye well, I will goe and cause hym to bee letten bloud, and kepe hym from slepe; then shall he bee purged to morowe in the mornyng. Bryng the pouder against the plague with you.

A constaunt man by his looke.[5]

A blacke sanctus.

Crispine.

God giue you good morowe, gentle maister *Auarus.* What, Master *Ambodexter?* how fare you both? Maister *Antonius* did[7] desire to haue spoken with you eight houres past. Indeede, within this two houres, sauyng your worshippes, hee hath taken a purgation, whiche hath[8] caste suche ayre abroade that I was not able to abyde in the chamber. I had forgotten my perfumes to make all well against your commyng.[9]

[1] Ed. 1564, "pretie" omitted. [2] Ed. 1564, haue. [3] Ed. 1564, hande.
[4] "he hath," &c., omitted in ed. 1564. [5] Ed. 1564, gesture.
[6] Ed. 1564, haue. [7] Ed. 1564, did moche. [8] Ed. 1564, haue.
[9] The words "against your commyng" are not found in ed. 1564.

Auarus.

What thinke you of hym? shall he escape or no? Who is with hym? I praie you tell mee and my brother *Ambodexter*.[1]

Crispine.

None but Doctor *Tocrub*,[2] whiche also desire your absence, because he hath[3] hym in cure, and trust to make hym sleepe after his lacke of rest, and to morow take your pleasure with hym.

Auarus.

Fare ye well: wee haue drawen and ingrossed his bookes; commende vs to Mayster Doctour. It were a good pastyme to take the footeclothe from his Mule for two or three howers in pastyme.

Ambodexter.

I had rather haue the Mule.

Auarus.

What the deuill doeth this doctor here? If this purging were not, we would clense and expulse with our resettes that whiche should serue our tourne well enough, by sweete Sainct Laurence.[4]

Ambodexter.

I warraunt you the doctour doth[5] make worke for vs both. We shall bryng our matters to passe in good tyme; take no care, manne, for the matter. Wee will preuente the doctour to morrow, when he commeth hether with a present, and bryng him some pretie thynges wherein *Antonie*[6] deliteth. We shall finde suche a[7] meanes to perswade with hym, by little and little, to bee Executours of his Will according to his old promise. Further, hee will take it kindly that wee doe claime kindred on hym by his mother's side, whiche was a kinde harted woman, and full of meritrix,[8] ha, ha, ha! She was in deede of those qualities; her sonne is like the mother as seemeth by one in the house, like Cowe like Calfe.[9]

---

[1] The words "and my brother Ambodexter," are not in ed. 1564.
[2] Ed. 1564, Capistranus.   [3] Ed. 1564, haue.
[4] The words "by sweete Sainct Laurence" do not occur in ed. 1564.
[5] Ed. 1564, doe.   [6] Ed. 1564, he.   [7] "a" omitted in ed. 1564.
[8] Ed. 1564, metrir.
[9] The words "like Cowe like Calfe" do not occur in ed. 1564.

Auarus.

I feare that damosell will marre altogether: she doeth rule the rost, she weares[1] the keies. He can neuer haue her out of his sight, yet Reinolde, his man, thinketh hymselfe in better[2] estimation with her then his master.

Ambodexter.

The last yere I counterfected a sickenes of purpose, as I can when I lust; I framed my Physicion to my phantasie, one master *Suilemob;*[3] no manne thought that I should haue liued two daies; when I was alone I laughed. You remember whom I made myne Executor, euen *Antonius*.[4] I then prouidently, by three thynges, did foresee this tyme and cause. The firste was his grate surfettes in banquetting; the second his watchyng at Chesse and Cardes; the thirde, you knowe what,[5] *Venus, Venus,* God wotte.

Auarus.

Well, well, be as may be[6] is no banning. I doe feare many thynges: Firste, the medicines may chaunce recouer hym, then shall we haue[7] nothyng. Well, Reinold and the damosell be euer in presence & watche hym; she cheares her maister with a louyng countenaunce; Reinolde saies that he hath doen true seruice a long tyme, &c. Well, I smell an other padde in the Strawe. When al this is doen the curate is a craftie knaue:[8] well can hee persuade and rehearse Gods vengeance, threates, & plagues, by examples most fearefull, like thonderboltes, describing the scalding house of hell, *ve, ve, ve,* with the story of *Diues* and *Pauper*, and the daie of iudgement; readyng the Homely of death, crying out, all is but vanite, vanitie and vexation of mynde, damnation except repentaunce and true confession from the harte and restitution of wronges; he will keepe a stirr and bryng our cousin into a fooles Paradise. It is hee that will raise vp all the beggers in the toune. He will crie, giue with your owne haude, for to day you are a man, to morowe earth and ashes; Dirige[9] helpe not in this case.

---

[1] Ed. 1564, ware. [2] Ed. 1564, more.
[3] The words "one master Suilemob" are not found in ed. 1564.
[4] Ed. 1564, Antonius Mantuanus.
[5] The sentence ends with the word "what" in ed. 1564.
[6] Ed. 1564, be as be maie. [7] Ed. 1564, wee shall haue.
[8] Ed. 1564, Rhetorician. [9] The words "Dirige," &c. are not found in ed. 1564.

Ambodexter.

First, let vs be sober and seeme to be sorrowfull for him, desiring nothyng but onely his life. If he stand in great daunger the doctor shall haue his leaue and tary no longer with hym, in whom I thinke hee hath[1] no hope to recouer; let hym be well rewarded. Secondlie, let Reinolde bee sente into the Countrie to the debitours[2] for money; tell hym it shall turne to his greate profite, and how his maister doeth intende to take hym as his sonne, and will truste none but onely hym to fetche the money in the countrey. Thirdly, I wil seeme to phantasie the minion, wishyng her to bee my wife, alledging what broken slepes she hath caused me to haue, and the causes[3] of my commyng hether onely for her staie. Then I will practise for the keies of the greate blacke chest, and of the steele casket. Fourthly, maister Curate shall be gently saluted with a Barnardes blowe; we will commende hym, we will praie with hym and also receive the Communion with our cousin, that he may haue a good opinion in vs; and deliuer hym a bagge with fiue pound in pence to giue to the poore, in whose absence peraduenture our Scribe and wee shall frame the wille. How like you this practise? If this will not serue I haue a shift of discant in store that I learned in Blosomes[4] Inne.

margin: A Craftie villaine.

Auarus.

The Deuill take altogeather so that we had the golde. Practise this, I praie you; you haue a good witte, by my troth. I could not sleape all this night for this matter; if you were not I could doe nothyng but stande like a sheepe. Oh,[5] his good, bolde cousin, that that, that.

Ambodexter.

I warrant you I haue had long experience in this trade. Every where within this realme I can doe the like with the helpe of *Periurus*,[6] whiche is a verie good pen man, cloase and honeste; he writeth sondrie handes, and is a liuely grauer of Seales hymself; also he[7] is a kinde harted felowe, for he will not sticke to lende his frende an othe if neede doe require.

margin: Pettifoggers fitte for the Pillerie.

---

[1] Ed. 1564, haue. [2] Ed. 1564, debtours. [3] Ed. 1564, cause.
[4] Ed. 1564, Bosomes. [5] This sentence is not found in ed. 1564.
[6] Ed. 1564, Avarus. [7] "he" omitted in ed. 1564.

Auarus.

The worlde is full of starting holes, men may scant knowe how to trust men now a daies; but for the goode reporte that I doe heare of this honest felowe I will bee glad to haue his acquaintance; I knewe diuers of his kinsmen thirtie[1] yeres ago. God haue mercie of all Christian soules! it was then a merie world, and will neuer bee so good againe vntill this Gospellyng Preachers haue a sweatyng sickness in Smithfielde and their Bible burnte. Well, would some were at libertie for their sakes. Well, well.

Ambodexter.

Oh, I doe remember that reuerent mortified father, that holy man, Bishop Boner, that blessed Catholike Confessour of Rome; if hee were againe at libertie he would not dallie to mocke[2] theim, but trimely woulde roste these felowes and after burne them: you knowe his workmanship verie well, a godly man.[3]

Auarus.

He is my cousin german, and *Periurus*, that honeste fellowe, was his boye,[4] and brought vp with him in his youth; Honest fellow.[5] and your Graundfather did penne his Prologue in the booke called *De Vera Obedientia*, when as they laughed merily, saiyng thei had rather put to their handes than either their heddes or hartes; wise men, wise men, by sainct Lambarte![6]

Ambodexter.

Yea, suche wisemen will serue the tyme, *Prudenter agere*, and bee as wise as Serpentes and simple as Doues.

Auarus.

To haue the nature of a Serpent I wil stande with them, but beshrowe my harte if I would be as simple as a Doue,[7] but rather as my good Lorde Boner, *Quasi Leo rugiens querens quem deuoret*. And thus he would expounde that text whiche muste haue suche a glose vpon it. As gentle as a Lion.[8]

---

[1] Ed. 1564, xx.   [2] Ed. 1564, make.
[3] The words "a godly man" do not occur in the 1st ed.
[4] Ed. 1573, doye.   [5] Eds. 1564, 1573, felowes.
[6] The words "by sainct Lambarte" are not found in ed. 1564.
[7] Ed. 1564 after "Doue," reads "either so simple, fearfull, or doltishe, but rather as," &c.   [8] This marginal note is not in ed. 1564.

Ambodexter.

I am alone vpon gloses, I haue arte in store to Sophist, I was brought vp 3 yere with a Frier of Mont Piller; he taught mee how to handle *prosa, obscurum, inordinatum,* and *barbarum*, with *genus* and *species.* Full well I can handle the matter, bothe *pro* and *contra.* Commonly these are the figures, and serue well to my purpose, as *Enigma, prœmiœ, ironiœ, sarcasimus, antephrasis,* and *charientismus.*[1] I have many rotten rules whiche do serue for the purpose;[2] I learned theim in Louen,[3] they are written in an old barbarous[4] booke. When wee are at more leasure I will shewe thee all my cunnyng, my gaines and profites. Nowe lette vs conferre both together this afternoone aboute our matters.

margin: Gloses.

Auarus.

Contented in that case; as for termes and trickes in Logike, I forse not of them, thei will paie for no horse bread. It is golde that maketh a gladde harte; he deserueth reuerence and rule that hath it and kept it. Goe, let vs dine together and sende for our friendes, *Rapax, Capax,* and *Tenax* to keepe vs compaignie an hower or twoo, for they are good fellowes, they haue kindred[5] through out all Englande.

margin: A good compaignie.

Ambodexter.

Agreed, I like their companie very wel, they are my frendes and kind harted men.

Auarus.

And mine[6] also. Go, let vs departe and not be seen muche together abroad, standyng in counsaile, because our matters are not curraunt; but[7] it shall be shortly, there are so many of the kindred.

Medicus.

Crispinus, where haue you been so long? I thought it a yeere since your departure, but I haue shortned[8] the tyme in beholdyng

---

[1] Eds. 1564, 1573, *chatientismus*.   [2] Ed. 1564, purse.
[3] Ed. 1564, at Paris; ed. 1573, at Louen.
[4] Ed. 1564, barbarous Frenche booke.
[5] The words "they haue kindred," &c., are not found in ed. 1564.
[6] This is the reading of ed. 1564. The later eds. give "And more also."
[7] The words "but . . kindred" are not found in ed. 1564.
[8] Ed. 1564, shorted.

this pitifull picture of *Lucretia* & this fearfull siege of Pauie. But this Mappe of the description of *Terra florida in America*[1] hath reioysed me; there the gold & precious stones and Balmes are so plentifull, siluer and spice are nothyng with them; no labour is in that land, long life they haue; one thing there is which liketh me not emong them.

Crispine.

What is that, maister Doctour?

Medicus.

They haue neuer sicknesse vntill death doe come; therefore there is no goode dwellyng for vs in suche a land. Further, it is saied that they haue no debate nor strife in their common wealthes.

Crispine.

Marie, then it is as vnprofitable for Lawiers as for Phisicians. I truste we shall neuer be in that case in this our countrie.

Medicus.

God defende vs from suche a Common wealthe, it would marre altogether. Now let vs go to the chamber doore and see how the worlde goeth with Master *Antonius*, and take our Phlebothomer with vs to let hym bloud.

Crispine.

I will waite on your maistership.

Medicus.

How doe you, good Maister *Antonius?* haue you taken any rest since I was with you?

Antonius.

No more, maister doctour, then if I had been laied on hot coales. Oh, sir, there was neuer manne in suche a case as I am in; I haue had moste fearefull dreames of theues to robbe mee. Me thought I was in the top of a high Tower, telling of money, and sodainly there came an yearthquake and shooke the Tower in peeces, and caste mee downe vpon weapons all bloudie, whiche a great nomber of Morians had in their handes; from them I fell in the fire, which was like high mountaines aboute mee, whereas

A Dreadfull case.

---

[1] Ed. 1578, Amricia.

was muche noyse and a cruell battaile. I did see there many
of myne olde acquaintaunce, whiche sometyme were of greate honour,
both men Spirituall and Temporall, and the Pope hymself, with
many of his frendes. They were in extreme wretchednesse, and
sore handled of fearefull monsters, and wormes gnawyng vppon their
breastes, vppon whom was written, Conscience hath accused me
and hell deuoured me, *Ve, ve, ve!* And thus I am tossed *A troubled*
to and fro. Alas, what shall I doe? Also I did heare *conscience.*
many ragged and sicke people crie vengeaunce on me, and men in
prison also, that said I had undoen them to inriche myself. Oh
good God!

Crispine.

Sir, I pray you let me herken in your eare.

Medicus.

What is the matter?

Crispine.

I will departe: his talke doeth so muche trouble mee; mee
thinke he doeth wounde my conscience. Also I will home, and
caste awaie a greate nomber of rotten drugges wherewith I haue
gotten muche money in deceiuyng the people. God forgiue mee!

Medicus.

The vicar of S. Fooles be your ghostly father. Are you so
wise? tary still with mee; let hym paie for your rotten drugges, for
I may saye to you that he is almoste rotten alreadie hymself; me
think your conscience is to much spiced with sodaine deuotion.

Antonius.

What meane you, master doctor, to wisper in the Apothecaries
eare?

Medicus.

Nothyng, sir; but I haue appoincted at what tyme that you
should receiue youre Clister, and how your Ptisante should bee
made, and in what order that your frontary should bee applied to
your forehed to cause you to sleape quietly. These dreames are
nothyng but proceading of the aboundance of choler, or els some
fearefull affection.[1] You are hot and drie, also the time is verie hotte;

---

[1] The words "or . . . affection" are omitted in ed. 1564.

the Sunne is now 20 degrees in Leo, the Dogge daies are to be obserued. Notwithstandyng, feare nothyng; I warraunt you, life for life, discomfort not your selfe, a man or a mouse.

Antonius.

You are a merie gentlemanne; doe your pleasure witn mee; I will put myselfe into your handes, I tell you. Hold, here is[1] twentie olde Angels that did see no Sonne this ten yere. Your Pothicarie shal be well considered; he semeth to be an honest man and a cunnyng fellowe; let hym sette vp all the boxes and glasses in the windowe, and put on his bonnette and sit doune there.[2]

Medicus.

What meane you, Sir? I pray you remember your self. So God helpe me, you are to blame. Well, I will not contrary you; my chief desire is to helpe you without the respect of money or gold or other of your commoditie. *Crispine*, set the boxes in the windowe; and you, Surgian, prepare your lace, staffe, and launce, Maister Wise,[3] with your vnce vesselles, that I may consider his bloud in order and due quantitie, for hether vnto hee is but in the augmentyng of his Feuer; further, he had no fitte this ten howers. Let hym bloud by little and little, and although he doe fall into *Lipothimion*, it is no matter; let hym bloudde vntill it partly doe chaunge into a good colour. Oh lorde! how might you liue if this bloud should haue remained any longer? Did you euer see the like? What a good harte he hath! the worst is paste; this would haue been a greate sore or Apostumation. Stop vp the vein a Gods name.

Wise.[4]

I did neuer see the like but once, whereas your maistership did a greate cure vpon a noble man, as I haue doen many, I thanke God and my cunnyng.[5]

Medicus.

Oh, are you aduised of that, M. Wise:[6] he is a good frende of

---

[1] Ed. 1564, are.
[2] The words "and sit doune there" are not found in ed. 1564.
[3] The marginal note is not in ed. 1564.   [4] Ed. 1564, Crispine.
[5] The words "as I . . . cunning" are omitted in ed. 1564.
[6] For "M. Wise" ed. 1564 reads "Crispine."

myne, I haue twentie pounde yerely of hym. He sente mee a fatte Bucke vpon mondaie last, and gaue me my Mule also, with a Veluet foote clothe. He[1] is well learned : he hath red the Apocalips.

Wise.[2]

Sir, when you sent me home I left your Mule standing at the doore; but as I returned I mette a Lackey clothed in Orenge Taunie and White, with a paire of bare tanned legges, and a blewe night cap with a plume of Fethers, ridyng on him as faste as he might gallop.

Medicus.

Oh, the passion of Christ! my Mule is stolen. I will hence; I had rather lose .xx. li.; I will tary no longer. My Mule! A great losse.[3] I will teach hym to ride on my Mule, I warrant hym.

Wise.[2]

Sir, he needeth no teachyng, he can ride well, I warrante you. I heard hym saie to a yonge man with a long cloke lined with yellowe, that his maister sent hym to cary a letter to a Marchaunte Venterer that was crossailed into *Terra Florida.*

Medicus.

Giue me my goune; fare ye well, Maister *Antonius;* as euil lucke as euer I had in all my life: my manne[4] is playing the knaue while my Mule is stolen.

Antonius.

I had thought the losse of your frend and of your Mule had not been bothe a like to you. What? for .xx. li.? I will paie it double; the knaue shal not escape. Wise[2] hath taken good markes vpon him. I will send to euery Warde, blinde lane, Innes, Wooddes, and fields after the villaine. I will take the matter on me because you come to me so gently; quiet your selfe, sit doune againe in the chaire; I were cast awaie if you wer gone, good maister Doctour Tocrub.[5]

---

[1] This sentence is not found in ed. 1564.   [2] Ed. 1564, Crispine.
[3] In eds. 1573, 1578, this marginal note is printed opposite Medicus' previous speech.
[4] The words "my manne," &c., do not occur in ed. 1564.
[5] Ed. 1564 omits "Tocrub."

Medicus.

I care not so much for the Mule, but that the gentleman[1] will take muche vnkindenesse, and thinke I should sette light by his gifte, and the Ruffians will laugh mee to skorne when they knowe howe I am handeled of the knaue boye. Well, I am contented with your offer. I praie you beware you slepe not; you shall suppe the thinne brothe of a Chicken by and by, made with the fower greate colde seedes and Cordial Hearbes. *Crispine,* I praie you make the brothe in some stone or siluer vessell; Copper or Brasse are not good for Maister *Antonius,* suche vessels are leprous.

Antonius.

If you wil haue it made of gold, you shal; I haue plentie, plentie.[2]

Medicus.

Wee shall make shifte with other thynges; golde shall serue to deaurate or gilde your Losenges, Electuaries, and *Manuschristi* withall.

Antonius.

Contented, so that it make on my side, whatsoeuer it bee. But mee thinke I feele sleepe approachyng: what shall I doe?

Medicus.

Drawe the Curtaines, open the luket[3] of the windowe, set Sallowes about the bed besprinkled with Vineger and rose water. Take of that hote mantle; let his head and shoulders bee bolstered vp; lye not on youre backe, leane towardes this side. Let vs talke together as[4] frendes: why are you so heauy and earthlike? God,[5] your colour is altered!

Antonius.

I must nedes I was made of earth. But where is the earth placed of whiche I was made, and of what fashion is it? Question.

Although I am of[6] the same, yet doe I stande in doubte of the matter.

---

[1] Ed. 1564 has "my lord" instead of "the gentleman."
[2] The words "I haue plentie, plentie" are not found in ed. 1564.
[3] Ed. 1564, luketts. [4] Ed. 1564, like.
[5] This sentence is not found in ed. 1564.
[6] Ed. 1564 has "walke vpon" instead of "am of."

Medicus.

The earth is moste heauie, and can be in no place but in the middest of heauen; not moueable, but round, and hangeth continually, about the whiche are the landes and countries of the world fixed, whiche *Aristotle* doth call *medium terræ, medium mundi.* Aristot. de cœlo & mundo.

Auarus.

Are there not bodies whiche are called simple? I haue heard saie so.[1]

Medicus.

Yes, forsoth, those are the fower: the fire hote and drie, the ayre hote and moyste, the water cold and moyste, the yearth cold and drie; and these are called the Elementes. The fower Elements.

Antonius.

Are there not bodies called mixed? what are they?

Medicus.

Animalia, as man, beast, fishe, foule, and wormes; *Vegetabilia,* as herbe, grasse, and Trees; and *Meneralia,* thynges under the yearth, as mettales. In the laste[2] matter I am verie connyng. Mixed bodies.

Antonius.

Lorde, how is this worlde staied?

Medicus.

The twoo Poles, *Articus* and *Artarticus,* Southe and Northe, are the extreme limites about whom the whole frame of heauen is wrapped, and is called *Axie cœli.*

Antonius.

Men say that certaine starres doe gouerne the thinges beneth here in yearth.

Medicus.

They doe so in deede, as it is wel proued, when as the Sunne and Moone doe enter into any of their circles in those greate bodies, then our little bodies in earth do feele the goodnes or euilnesse of them,

---

[1] The words "I haue heard saie so" are not in ed. 1564.
[2] The words "In the laste," &c. are not in ed. 1564.

as *Aries*, *Leo*, and *Sagittarius* are hot, drie, and bitter, Cholerike, and are gouernyng hot and drie thinges, and this is called the fierie triplicitie. The seconde triplicitie is of ayre, hot and moyste, sanguine, sweete, and doe gouerne Sanguine people. An other triplicitie is of water, cold and moiste, Flegmatike, hauyng the gouernment of cold rawe bodies. The laste is the yearth, the mother of all thinges, colde and drie, Melancholie.

Antonius.

What doe the knowledge of these thynges profite to Phisicke, I praie you tel me?

Medicus.

Most chiefly, for where as the Philosopher doth leaue, there the Phisition doth begin; that is, he must be first a good natural Philosopher, he must haue the knowledge of tymes and seasons, and bee acquainted with complexions of men, obseruyng the nature of thynges, and the climates vnder heauen, with the course of the Sunne, Moone, and Starres, ayre and diet, &c. A greate matter.[1]

Antonius.

I pray you, is there a soule in man?

Medicus.

Yea, forsothe.

Antonius.

Why, then there must needes be a greater thing as the cause of euery liuyng soule, which I take to be God, which hath made all thynges; and when you and I talked together you seemed that *Non est deus.* God.

Medicus.

I professed to followe *Aristotle*, but my meanyng was that I credite not the Bible matters; I am no Diuine, I finde no reasons there for my tourne, they are to harde thynges for me; I commende them to *Darbel* and *Duns*, &c.

Antonius.

Why, doeth *Aristotle* shewe any better reasons than is in the Bible? Then I pray you what is the power of the soule?

[1] Not in ed. 1564.

Medicus.

In the soule, saieth *Aristotle* in his booke of *Ethiques*, he[1] hath three sundrie powers. The one is named vegitable, in whiche euery man taketh part with herbes, trees, and plantes. The seconde part of the soule is named sensible: in this parte manne and beaste are bothe a like in mouyng, &c. The thirde parte is more whiche is rationall or hauyng reason, and this parte of reason hath bothe acte to do well and power to doe euill. And these two are called *Intellectiue*, whiche learneth, descerneth, and judgeth in eury thyng that may be seen, felt, heard, or vnderstanded; but the power vnreasonable, as sodaine raging, crying, &c., is ascribed vnto the Lion, Horse, Hogge, &c. How like you this maner of talke? yet here is no Scripture But Aristotle, I assure you.

The three powers of[2] the soule.

Antonius.

Then it should appeare that the soule hath vertues: howe many, I praie you?

Medicus.

The first vertue is called *Intellectual*, from whiche springeth wisedome, Science, and prudence. And the seconde is called morall, whiche is the mother of many good thynges, as chastitie, liberalitie, humanitie, and good maners.

Antonius.

What is the cause of these two vertues in the soule?

Medicus.

The vertue Intellectuall engendereth and is nourished by learnyng of good tutours and men of experience, or readyng of good bokes of Philosophie, which is a secret vertue in the soule. And also the morall commeth by good custome, and not by nature, as if one manne had two soonnes, the one brought vp in keepyng cattell, the other in daiely learnyng good lessons, although nature did frame their bodies in like shape,[3] yet they should not bee like in conditions. Morall prouideth that naturall thynges in them bothe can not be moued by contrarie custome. For stones naturally, though they be cast neuer so high by arte, yet must they naturally

Example.

---

[1] Ed. 1564, it. [2] Ed. 1564, partes.
[3] Eds. 1564, 1573, like in shape.

fall doune againe. Euen so of fire, beyng driuen doune, yet it will cast his flames vpwarde; so vertue is not in vs by nature, but onely by power to receiue theim, for euery thyng that is in vs by nature, first it is[1] by power, and after commeth to act as it commeth to the senses of mankinde. For none can deny but first man hath power to heare, see, feele, &c. So the power doth preuent and commeth before the act in nature. *A good note.*[2]

Antonius.

Then if power goeth before the act, then a man is called honeste, good, or chaste, before either honestie,[3] goodnesse, or chastitie appeareth in hym.

Medicus.

In thynges morall euermore the acte goeth before the power. An example: a schoolmaister is called a teacher because of his learnyng, whiche is the woorke goyng before the power. And the cause of a good man is his goode workes, and so of the euill, whose woorke is either dronkennesse, adulterie, thefte, &c., they make hym euill.

Antonius.

Then it should appeare that this thyng called *actus* or worke bringeth vertue and vice in man.

Medicus.

What els? doeth not euery man that liueth eate? But if he eate to muche or to little, doth it not bryng sicknesse. Euen so of to muche labour or idlenesse, of to muche boldnesse or cowardnesse, are not these actes vicious and euill? And dooeth not one meane moderate theim bothe? Extreames are euer hurtfull.

Antonius.

What remedie then, I praie you?

Medicus.

Nothyng is better than a meane called temperaunce, whiche is gouerned by Prudence, whiche is euer content betwene both, and reioyseth in it. *Temperance.*

---

[1] Ed. 1564 has "first it is in vs by powers." [2] Not in ed. 1564.
[3] Ed. 1564, nonestie.

Antonius.

So then if a man fell into extreame aduersitie, and sustaine it paciently in his sicknesse, pouertie, or cause of grief, calle you this a meane or no? <small>Aduersitie.</small>

Medicus.

In euery woorke or sufferyng there is pleasure or displeasure. If a man do reioyce in trouble, in chastitie, in bearyng of cruell woordes or slaunder, the same is a prudent man, and his sufferyng maketh it a meane to hym. But other men that are chastised and will suffer outwardly, and it greeueth theim in so doyng; the same is vicious, and laketh meane or prudence. <small>Prudence.</small>

Antonius.

Hath the soule any delites in her or no?

Medicus.

Yes, truely, in three thynges. The firste profitable, whereof springeth housbandrie to nourishe the yearth, as also Phisicke to help the body, knighthod to go to battel, &c. The seconde is delectable, as takyng pleasure in thynges doen, whiche is chiefly nourished of the soule, in whiche consisteth all the pleasures of the worlde. The thirde is called good, that is, to be verteous, louing, sober, pacient; and also to the soule or minde are enioyned habite, power, and passion. <small>Profite.</small> <small>Pleasure.</small> <small>Virtue.</small>

Antonius.

Haue yong children the soule in all poinctes as women haue or no, in operation or election?

Medicus.

Aristotle saith that operation of the will of the soule is common to children, but the election or choyce be not in them to will.

Antonius.

What is will in the soule?

Medicus.

The will is the intent, but election is the antecedent to the intent, for election goeth before operation or worke, and the woorke doeth folowe the same, as doyng of thynges, buying, sellyng, and all the artes and sciences are so to be considered. First by election, then by operation; as by arte I do proue you to haue the pestilence; experience hath taught mee, whiche yong children can not knowe, as Grammer, Rhetorick, Music, Phisicke, before they haue learned them or begon with their principles. *First election, then operation.*

Antonius.

Now I will stop and laie a strawe, and comen as yet no more of the matters of the soule, but onely of the bodie, and namely in this poincte of the Pestilence. What is the cause of the same, good maister doctour? *Pestilence.*

Medicus.

That which we do see we do testifie, and that whiche we do testifie is true. Therefore no man ought in matters whiche appertaineth to the estate of life to write fables or lyes, but that whiche is of great aucthoritie and of good experience. The[1] Pestilent feuer, saieth *Hypocrates*, is in twoo partes considered; the first is common to euery man by the corruption of the[2] ayre; The second is priuate or particular to some men through euill diete, repletion, whiche bringeth putrifaction, and finally mortification. And *Galen*, in the differences of Feuers, doeth affirme the same, saying, *Vnam aerem viciatum ac putridum, alteram humores*[3] *corporis vitioso*[4] *victu collectos et ad putriscendum paratos.* *Auicen* also, *Tractus quartus de febribus pestilentialibus, Cap. i.* When there doth come a sodaine alteration or change in the qualitie of water from Colde to heate, or transmutation from sweetenesse to stincke, as it chaunceth in waters through corrupted mixture of putrified vapours[5] infectyng bothe ayre and water, whiche of their owne simplicitie are cleane, but through euill mixture are poysoned; or when stronge Windes doe carrie pestilent fume or vapours from stinkyng places to the cleane partes, as bodies dead of the Plague vnburied, Or mortalitie in battaile, death of cattell, rotten Fennes, commyng sodainly by the impression of

The cause of the Pestilence.
Hypocrates de flatibus.
Galen libri i. de differentiis Feb. Cap. v.
Aetius de re Medica, lib. 5. Paulus, libri 2.
Rasis in lib. de pest. Gale. lib. i. De Diffe. Fe. cap. iiii.

---

[1] Ed. 1564, This. [2] Omitted in ed. 1564. [3] Old eds., homoree.
[4] Eds 1564 1573, *virioso.* [5] Ed. 1564, vapour.

aire, creepyng to the harte, corruptyng the spirites, this is a dispersed Pestilence by the inspiration of the[1] ayre. Also by repletion, Venus, Bathyng, or opening the poures, rotten foode, fruite, much wine, or immoderate labour, or the tyme beyng hotte and moyste. These are greate causes.

Antonius.

At what tyme of the yere dooth the Pestilence cast forthe her poyson?

Medicus.

In the time of Haruest, saieth *Hypocrates*, are most sharpe and deadly sicknesses, but lesse daunger in the Spryng tyme; and in the tyme of sundrie chaunge of windes, when the weather is hotte and moyste. Hyp. Aph. xix.

Antonius.

To what persones, I praie you, doeth the Pestilence come?

Medicus.

Moste chiefly to theim vnder the place infected, then to sluttishe, beastly people, that keepe their houses and lodynges vncleane, their meate, drinke, and clothyng moste noysome, their laboure and trauaile immoderate; or to theim whiche lacke prouident wisedome to preuente the same by good diete, ayre, medicine, &c.; or to the bodies hotte and moyste; and these bodies do infect other cleane bodies, and whereas many people doe dwell on heapes together, as *Auecen* saieth, *Et communicat multitudine homimum*, &c., Fen. I. Tract. IIII.

Antonius.

By what signe or token is this perilous plague or stripe of the pestilence best knowen emong the Phisitions? Goe not about the bushe with subtile wordes, but plainely speake the truthe to me, beyng in this fearfull daunger as you do wel knowe that I am in.

Medicus.

The signes are moste manifest, whiche are the starres running course or rase after their causes. Oh, the most fearefull Eclipses of the Sunne and Moone, those heauenly bodies, are manifest signes of the pestilence emong men, and the starres Causes and signes of pestilence.

---

[1] Omitted in ed. 1564.

cadente in the beginnyng of Haruest or in the moneth of September; or muche Southe Winde or Easte winde in the *Canicular* daies, with stormes and cloudes, and verie colde nightes and extreame hotte daies, and muche chaunge of weather in a little time; or when birdes do forsake their egges, flies or thinges bredyng vnder the ground do flie high by swarmes into the ayre, or death of fishe or cattell, or any dearth goyng before, these are the signes of the Pestilence and euident presages of the same.

Antonius.

These are good signes general; but particular, what[1] manifest tokens do signifie the Plague or Pestilence in a mannes owne proper bodie?

Medicus.

They which are smitten with this stroke or plague are not so open in the spirits as in other sicknesses are, but straite winded; they do swone and vomite yellowe cholour, swelled in the stomacke with muche paine, breaking foorth with stinking sweate; the extreme partes very cold, but the internall partes boiling with heate and burning; no rest; bloud distillyng from the nose, Vrine somwhat watrie and sometyme thick with stincke, sometyme of colour yellowe, sometyme blacke; scaldyng of the tongue; ordure most stinckyng; with red eyen, corrupted mouthe, with blacknesse, quicke pulse and deepe but weake, headache, altered voyce, losse of memorie, sometyme with ragyng in strong people. These and suche like are the manifeste signes howe the harte hath drawne the venome to it by attraction of the ayre, by the inspiration of the arters to the hart, and so confirming it to be the perilous feuer pestilentiall. This is most true, of this commeth foule *bubo*,[2] *antaxis* and *Carbuncles*, Sores through putrifaction, as *Galen* saieth: *li. iii. De presage, Auicen Fe. i. tract ii.*,[3] *Galen, lib. i. De Diffe.* cap. iiii. *Et Rasis de constitutione pestilentiæ ad Mansorem*. Also this feuer is scant to bee recoured and almost past help when these *Symptomatas* do appeare, as Galen saith, iii. *De præsage expul, qua propter neque*[4] *hos curare tentandum erit.*

Ruff. Auleto fatetur. Aetius. Cap. xcv. Libr. v., viii. Paulus, Libri i. cap. xxxv.

[1] Ed. 1573, but what, [2] Ed, 1564, bubos.
[3] Ed. 1564, iiii; ed. 1573, iii. [4] Ed. 1573, *neq.*

Antonius.

You haue declared vnto me a fearefull tale of the Plague, whereof[1] thousandes haue and shall die. A pitifull case how it commeth emong people sodainly, euen as you haue shewed the cause primatiue in the ayre;[2] the antecedent when the same ayre is drawen into the harte by attraction of the arters; the coniuncte when it with boyling heat doth chaunge by putrifaction nature into the worse parte; and almost past cure of any phisicion when it is come to this point, as I gather by your late talke, which doth put me in greate feare of my life. But I will comen[3] with you for others whiche are not infected; howe may they bee moste safely defended, maister doctour? *Primatiue, antecedent, coniuncte causes of the Pestilence.*

Medicus.

Would you faine knowe? Surely I wil declare thee the beste defence that I can; I will hide nothyng. First of all, let all men, women, and children auoide out of the euill ayre into a good soyle, and then, accordyng to their age, strength of nature, and complexion, let euery one of them with some good medicine drawe from the bodie superfluous moysture, and diminish humour, hotte and drie, and vse the regiment of diet to dryng, sharped with vineger or tart thynges, and lesser meates; not so much wine as they haue vsed in custome; neither Potage, Milke, vnripe fruites, hotte Spices, Dates, or Honie, or sweete meates, wine with Suger, are not tollerable; no anger or perturbations of the mynd, specially the passion called feare, for that doth drawe the spirites and blood inwards to the hart, and is a very meane to receiue this plague; neither vse actes venerous, nor bathyng, either with Fume, stoue or warme water, (for this cause)—they all doe open the pores of the bodie; neither quaffyng or muche drinkyng. Euen so thirste or drinesse is not tollerable, or immoderate exercise or labour, specially after meate. Music is good in this case, and pleasaunt tales, and to haue the meates well sauced *Good aire. Gale. de ter. 1 ad Pito. Cap. xvi. Paul. li. ca. xxxvi. Avicen de preser. a peste, fen.[4] li. tract iiii. Rasis ad almon. libr. de pest. Cap. ii. Trouble of mind or fear. A goodly rule against the Plague.*

---

[1] Ed. 1573, whereof a.   [2] Ed. 1564, thaire.
[3] Ed. 1564, common (*i. e.* commune).   [4] Ed. 1573, sen a tract. 4.

with cleane sharpe vineger. Forget not to keepe the chamber and clothyng cleane, no Priuies at hand, a softe fire with perfumes in the mornyng. Shifte the lodging often time, and close in the Southeaste windowes,[2] specially in the tyme of mistes, cloudes, and windes; And vse to smell vpon some pleasaunt perfume, And to bee letten bloud a little at once, and to take Pilles, *contra pestem:* that is a good preseruative against the plague.

A goodly medicine for the sore.[1]

Note also that clisters are good before the opening of veines.

Antonius.

These are good rules, & happie are they that doe wisely obserue them in time, place, and maner accordingly; but if one be newly infected, what remedie then, as when a man is sicke, and the sore appereth not?

Medicus.

A commyng forthe like a *Bubos* are signes of those partes from whiche they doe swel; as example, in the left side, head, neck, flanckes, &c. But often tymes the Plague sore will not appere; the very cause is this: Nature is to weake, and the poyson of the infection to strong that it can not be expelled, and this is moste perilous of all, when such a cruell conquerour doth raigne within the harte, the principall part of life, nowe possessed with death. The causes of this I haue declared before, with signes to the same; notwithstanding, consider two thinges: first, whether it is in bodies Sanguine and Cholerike, or theim whiche are Flegmatike or Melancholie, or not. The firste twoo, bloud is the cause, the seconde twoo aboundaunce of euill humours. Therefore let blood, where as it hath the victorie, and purge wheras other humours hath pre-domination or chief rule: in some men that haue verie stronge bodies, firste purge, then let bloud. Note this: that what side be infected let blood on that side; if it be aboue the hedde, open *Cephalica;* if it be vnder the armes, *Basilica*, or harte veine; if it be aboute the throte, then open *Melleola;* about the flankes, bealie, legges, &c., open *Iecoriaria.* If thei are verie weake or yong, then boxyng is good to the necke,

Libri Epid. Sect. II. Apho. iiii.

Consider two speciall thynges.

Avicen. Curati. Febri. Pesti. li. iiii. Fen. i. tract iiii.

Leo. Actus de medend, mor. Libri iiii.

---

[1] Not in ed. 1564.   [2] Ed. 1564, windes.

shoulders, backe and thighes; if the stomacke be full, then with speed vomet, and these thinges drawe the venome from the hearte and remoue the poison.

Antonius.

This is good in the cure of the Pestilence, for I dooe praise this blood lettyng verie well in the beginnyng of the sicknesse.

Medicus.

Blood must be letten in the beginnyng of the sickenesse. For example, like as a pot is clensed of the scumme or fome <small>Example.</small> in the beginning when it plaieth on the fire, and thereby the liquor is cleansed within the potte, euen so blood lettyng and pilles doe helpe and cleanse the Pestilence when it beginneth firste to boile within the bodie. Howbeit, certaine people maie <small>Who maie not not bleede, as women whiche haue their times abound- be letten blood.</small> auntlie, or menne hauing fluxe of the Hemoroides, children verie young, or people weake and aged.

Antonius.

I praie you what quantitie of blood must be letten?

Medicus.

Forsoth, fower vnces, or little more, and must bee doen euery moneth, sometyme in the *Median*, sometyme in the <small>Quantitie of *Basilica*, &c., And not to slepe after the same during blood letten.</small> six, seuen, or eight howers.

Antonius.

What Pilles doo you vse againste the Plague?

Medicus.

The beste Pilles generallie vnder heauen, and is thus made. Take the beste Yellowe Aloes, twoo vnces, Myrrhe and <small>Ruff. contra Saffron, of eche one vnce, beate them together in a pest., Avicen. libri iiii. Fen. 1, Morter a good while, putte in a little sweete wine, then tract iiii. Paul, Libri ii. Cap. rolle it vp, and of this make fiue Pilles, or seuen of one xxxvi.</small> dragme; whereof take eurie daie next your harte a Scruple or more, it will expulse the Pestilence that daie, &c.

Antonius.

Haue you anie good potion in store for the Pestilence, to be dronke a morninges when the Pilles are not taken?

Medicus.

None better than this: take *Theriaca*, of the making of *Andromachus*, ij Scruples, whiche is a Triacle incomperable, passyng againste bothe poison and Pestilence; and the *Antidotari*[1] of *Mithridatis* 1 Scruple; bole Amoniacke, prepared, half a Scruple; and of the water of distilled Roses, Scabious and Buglosse, of eche one vnce, mingled together. But this Medicine muste be had of *Crispine*, or one of his companions, which vse no rotten ware.

<small>Galenus, libri ix. de simplic.</small>

<small>Fuch. de Mede. morbis, libri iiii.</small>

Antonius.

Haue you any good pouder?

Medicus.

One better, I assure you, then a kinges raunsome, and thus it must be made: take the leaues of *Dictamnus*, and the rootes of Turmentill, of Pimpernell, of Seduall, of Gentian, of Betonie, of eche halfe an vnce; bole Armoniacke, prepared,[2] an vnce; *Terra Sigellata*, iij dragmes; fine Aloes & Myrrhe, of eche half an vnce; Safron, a dragme; Masticke, ij dragmes: beate them together finely and searsed. This is the pouder: of this must a dragme be dronke in iiij or vi sponfull of Rose or Sorell water, when danger approacheth, or in the tyme of danger.

Antonius.

These ar strong thinges for many weke stomakes: is there any other holsom thinges?

Medicus.

The sirrupes of Violettes, of Sorell, of Endiue, of sower Limondes, of eche like, mingled with Burrage water, and a Ptisane made of Barlie mingled together, is verie holsome to drinke: put in the pouder of bole Armoniack, whiche is of a singular vertue to coole; for Galen did help thousandes at Rome with the same Bole and the *Theriaca* mingled together, in a greate pestilence. But in the pesti-

---

[1] Eds. 1573, 1578, *antridotari*.   [2] Eds. 1573, 1578, Armoniackle.

lence tyme, one beyng infected therewith, let hym sweate by warme thinges, as hot tiles, &c.; and let not the pacient eate, sleepe, or[1] drinke; and eate light meates, as Henne, Capon, Cheken, Partriche, eating often and little at once, with sause made sharpe of veneger, Oringes, sharpe Limondes, or Sorel; and in the first day of the sickenes, that the pacient bee kept from sleepe by talkyng, sprinklyng of swete water, rubbyng of the bodie, as nose, eares, or[2] soft pullyng of the eares, as thei may be suffered, or a Sponge dipped in Vineger applied to the nose; and if vehement drinesse or heate dooeth approache, then drinke the Syruppes laste rehearsed, and haue the chamber cleane kepte, and also parfumed fower tymes of the daie. Beware of stincke; let the perfumes be made with *Olibanum*, Mastike, wood of Alooes, Benjamin, Storax, *Laudanum*, Cloues, Iuniper, or suche like, and sprincle all the chamber about with vineger; roses in the windowes, or greene braunches of Sallowe or of Quinces are good, sprinkled with Rose water and Vineger.[3]

Antonius.

I haue heard saie that Garlike and newe Ale shoulde be good for the Plague.

Medicus.

You doe saie truthe. Garlike is good for to bryng it, but not against it: it is so hotte, and hath power attractiue, and that is verie euill, and a meane to bryng the plague; so are Onions, Leekes, Rocket, Radishe, and suche baggage whiche are solde about in curie streate in Plague[4] tyme as meanes for to bring the same; it is pittie to suffer suche thinges. Furder, the multitudes of infected people emong the whole infecting them, or wearyng the apparell of the dedde bodies of the Pestilence, whiche should bee burned; for it is like a fire whan it hath gotten the victorie, and can not bee quenched. Priuies, filthie houses, gutter chanilles,[5] uncleane kept; also the people sicke goyng abrode with the plague sore running, stinkyng, and infectyng the whole; or vnwise, rashe, passing with an emptic stomake out of the house.

Good observations.

---

[1] Ed. 1564, nor.   [2] Eds. 1573, 1578, of.
[3] Ed. 1564 adds in the margin, "Avicen, libr. iiii. Fen. 1. Tract iiii. Ras."
[4] Ed. 1564, Plaguie.   [5] Ed. 1564, gutters, chanilles.

Neither to sitte tipplyng and drinking all the daie long, nor vse runnyng, wrestlyng, Daunsyng, or immoderate labour, whiche dooe onely[1] open the pores, but also cause the winde to bee shorte, and the pulses to quicke, and the arters drawe to the harte when it panteth, the pestilenciall ayre and poyson. And what is worse than feare of minde, when one doeth heare ill tydyng, the death of the[2] father, mother, child, &c.? By it the spirites and blood are drawen inwardes to the harte. Also of care, anger, wrath, &c.: these are al perilous.[3] Mirth must be vsed specially in this case. Cattes, Dogges, Swine, Duckes, Doues, Hennes, or Gese are very vn- holsome nere vnto the place or mansion of dwellyng, or lye dedde in diches nere the towne; or many people lying together in one bedde; or longe watchyng in the night; or costifuesse of the bealie. Shut vp the hot house doores and tennis plaie, whiche are moste venemous. Be neuer without the electuarie of nuttes, thus made: cleane Whalnuttes xx, fatte Figges xiij, herbe Grace two handfull, of Worme wodde, Fetherfu, or rather Cotula Fætida, called *Buphthalmus*, called Oxe eye, and Scabios, of eche one handfull, the rootes of *Aristolochia longa* halfe an vnce, *Aristolochia rotunda* an vnce and a halfe, The rotes of Turmentill and of the lesser Burre called *Petasitus*, Pimpernell, of eche ij vnces and a halfe, the leaues of the berie[4] Dictamini one handful, Bay beries iij Dragmes, the pouder of Hartes horne twoo drames and a halfe, Maces, Myrrrhe, Bole Armoniacke, and the yearth of Limondes,[5] of eche Dragmes three, Salt of the Sea a dragme and a halfe, *Nux vomica* dragmes twoo, Buglos flowers one handfull, stamped together by arte & with clarified honie make it; this is good to be eaten a dragme euerie mornyng. Forget not the Pilles of *Ruffi:* of them maie be taken one at once.

The best remedie, the worst meane.

Fuch lib. iiii. de morb. Electuarii de Nucibus.

Antonius.

After or with this Pestilence there wil a fearefull sore appere, as we haue the knowledge vniuersall by painefull experience, whiche we dooe call the plague sore. What doe you saie to the same sore?

---

[1] Eds. 1564, 1573, not onely.   [2] Omitted in ed. 1564.
[3] Ed. 1573, perious.   [4] Eds. 1564, 1578, verie.
[5] Ed. 1564, Limodes.

Medicus.

This sore is called *Carbunculus*, of Carbo a Cole, or *Anthrax*, they are bothe one and not twoo, and is ingendered of moste sharpe hotte and grosse blood, whiche nature doeth cast forthe through the skinne to one particular part with extreme paine and perille to the bodie, whose Primatiue cause was the corruption of aire or diete drawen to the harte, of whiche pestiferous smoke or poisoned fume this sore hath his cause, & the same sore is the effect followyng. *[Carbo & Anthrax are one.]*

Antonius.

What are the signes when it commeth nere hande?

Medicus.

A feuer going before, noisome and lothesomenesse of stomacke, wambelyng of the harte, pulse not equall, vrine stinking, desirous of slepe, perilous dreames with startyng through the sharpnesse of hotte and burnyng humours; and then a litle pushe will creepe forth like a scabbe, sometyme more then one, then it will increase, and shine like pitche or *Bytumen* with passyng pain, and then it will haue a crust like vnto the squames or flakes of Iron when thei fall of when the Smith doeth worke, and in colour like ashes is this cruste wrought by extreme heate and burnyng, therefore it maie be called the burnyng Cole or *Ignem persicum*. Furder, there are fower colours to bee obserued in the sore besides the crust: yelowe, redde, grene, and blacke. The first twoo are not so daungerous as the seconde twoo are. Yet, saieth *Rasis*, in his book of the Pestilence, to *Mansor* the king, that the Carbuncle is deadlie and most perillous. And *Auicen* affirmeth the blacke to be incurable, specially when a feuer Pestilence doe reigne. Sometyme it is drawen backe againe into the bodie, then no remeadie. Sometyme it happeneth in the most noble places, as nere the harte, the throate, moste perilous, with sodaine stopping the spirites of life. *[Signs of the Plague. Where the plague sore is placed.]* Some pestilent sores do come in the clensing places, as arme holes, flanckes, &c. And when nature is so stronge to caste it forthe with a redde colour, palishe or yellowishe, the cure is not then verie harde.

Antonius.

It should seeme to bee moste harde. You haue shewed more perilles then helpes bee therevnto :[1] but if there be any remedies, what are thei? I praie you tell them, for in that poincte you maie doe muche good.

Medicus.

Euen as I haue rehearsed before so will I againe begin in the cure of the carbuncle, of the openyng of a veine ; and if none other thyng doe let, as extreme weakeness, &c., then let the pacient bleede vntill the defection of the spirites, or nerehande swonyng. Let it bee doen on that side greued or afflicted, as I haue saied before in the feuer Pestilence of the Mediane, &c. Also forget not eight speciall thinges. First the substaunce, as compasse, lengthe, depthe, hardnesse, &c. Second, the matter wherof it is bredde, as blood, &c. The thirde as accidente through the dolor, as a feuer, rednesse, &c. Fowerth, to knowe it from a cause, whereof a doubte mighte arise thereof. And this is the difference betwene theim : a Carbuncle in the beginnyng is verie harde, flamyng redde, extreme paine, &c., as I haue saied before, and will come quickelie to his hedde. But *Cancer* is not so redde, neither so painefull, yet muche harder, and longer tyme or it commeth to the head. But when it beginneth to waxe softe, then it ripeth faster then the Carbuncle. The fifte of the causes efficient, whether it bee ripe through concoction or no, or the qualities of the corrupted humours, or hardnesse, &c. The sixt in what place it is, in place of perill or no. The seuenth is to woorke by incision, plaster, &c. The viii is good diet, as aire, meate, drinkes, slepe, &c. These are verie good obseruations worthie of memorie in this case. And now foloweth a perill to the *Chirurgian*, which must be richly rewarded, for he putteth his life in daunger in that, that he helpeth the sore bodie infected ; hee ought to be prouident that doth take this matter in hand, and before he cometh to the pinch to eate his *antidotarie* of *Metridatum*, or to haue a sponge with strong vinegar applied to his nosthrelles to arme hymselfe against the poisoned aire ;

<small>Gal. attributus alter dinamidis. To know the Anthrax from the Cancer.</small>

<small>A caviate for the Chyrurgian.</small>

---

[1] Ed. 1564, hether vnto.

and to take his launce in his hand accordyng to the art, taking heede
that in launcyng he cutte no vaine or Senewe whiche haue societie
with eche other, therefore launce not verie depe. This is no straunge
thing after bloodlettyng, to launce the sore to let forthe the matter.
In some it will come forthe aboundauntlie when it is ripe or rotten;
in other some not, because the humours are grosse and baken together,
or the runnyng matter farre in or skant ripe, and nothyng will come
forthe but Salte, sharpe, filthie, stinckyng water. Then beware of
any thing that might driue it backe againe into the bodie, as colde,
bole armen, &c.; then thinsicion must be made in the lowest place,
so that thereby the matter maie the soner auoide, and muste be made
in the forme croked, if it bee not in a place full of senewes; if it be,
then make the insicion long; after the matter is run forth then couer
it with lint dipped in this followyng, which is excellent good, yea,
if the matter be stubborne in the sore. Take Quinse <small>Note this well.</small>
seede, Galles, of eche iij Dragmes, Myrrhe, *Olibanum*, and Aloes,
of eche ij Dragmes and halfe, Alom ij dragmes, *Aristologia* the round
rootes, *Calamenthe* as muche, Calamenthe i dragme and a halfe,
Calcanthum a scruple, all beaten finelie; then temper it together in a
little Redde Wine made in small rolles. You maie kepe them drie,
and then in this case disolue it, or part of it, in the water of stilled
milke; applie this with lint into the sore, also in this case to washe
the sore with a sponge dipped in the warme waters of <small>To washe the</small>
dragones, Scabious, swete wine, Arristologia, and *Com-* <small>place.</small>
phori, or their decoction, And to haue the rootes of *Comphori*, of
Lillies, of Mallowes sodden in white wine vntill they be softe, then
stamped and drawen through a strainer; put thereunto barly meale &
honie of roses.[1] This is a verie good thyng to applie to the sore after
the washing for iij[2] hours, and will digest it. An other <small>A good medicine</small>
good medicen both to ripe and assuage the pain: mallowes, <small>to ripe.</small>
violets, camomile, of eche halfe an handfull, Dill half as much;
seeth them and bray them, then ad to them barly meale & oyle of
roses, flax sede, beane meale, of eche iij vnces. Seeth them in swete
wine vntill they waxe thicke and make plaister; and to the places

---

[1] Ed. 1564 has in margin, "a good medicen for the sore."
[2] Ed. 1564, xij.

aboute the rootes of the carbuncle round about it, this is good both
to eradicate & defend the same. Seeth fower oringes in vinegar or sorell, and put a little bole armin to it, dip a cloth or flaxe in it, and applie it round about the sore; manie tymes renewe it in this cure, reade M. Thomas Gailes worthie booke. And to take awaie the harde crust of the carbuncle doe this.[2] Take ceruse, Vermilion sublimated, of eche iij dragmes, beaten finely in pouder; and part of this maie bee cast vpon the same. And to this maie folow mallowes, violetes, lettes, of eche one handfull sodden in mutton brothe, the yolkes of three egges, barlie meale, oile of roses, and freshe butter, of eche three vnces. This plaister applied on will take awaie the Pestilent crust; also the emplastrum of *Diachilon paruum*, twoo vnces, with *Amoniake* and *Galbanum*, of eche one vnce, made in a plaister applied to the place, or a plaister of figges. Doues doung and Vallerian rootes and one[3] roote of Mallowes, made and applied vpon the sore are verie good ripers, and do muche preuaile in this cure; and, further, to bryng the cicatrice if need require. Take oile of Myrrhe, of roses, of violettes, of eche two vnces; shepes Tallowe three vnces, gottes tallowe one vnce and a halfe, Juice of Colewortes three vnces; seeth them together softlie vntill the iuice bee consumed, then putte thereunto halfe an vnce of Vermilion, ceruse as muche, and ij Dragmes of letherge of Gold, and seeth them vnto a blacknes, stirre theim with a sticke, then put to theim six vnces of[4] Turpentine, and as muche waxe as shall suffice to make it in the forme of a cærot. And this will make a strong cicatris; and when the matter hath runne muche, and is paste venim, then this is a powder moste precious to caste in and drie it up little & little: take ashes of Dyll, of burnt leade, of *Terra* lemnia, of eche one dragme; litharge of siluer, flowers of pomgarnates, and galles without holes, of eche two dragmes; ceruse, Creuishelles, snailes hornes, roche Alom burnt, of eche ij scruples beaten in powder; this is the powder. And hereafter followeth a good ointmente to heale the sore. Oile of

---

[1] Ed. 1564, M. Gaile. [2] Ed. 1564, thus. [3] Ed. 1564, the rootes.
[4] Ed. 1578, omitted in ed. 1564. [5] Ed. 1564, an.

Roses ij vnces, Ceruse, burnt leade, Litharge, of eche one a scruple; red Roses ij scruples in powder, the rootes of the greate *Comphori*, and the flowers of Pomegranates, bole Armen of eche one scruple, the seede of Purslen twoo graines, white waxe asmuche as shall suffice; and make this ointmente in a Leaden Morter if it maie be. Emong al simple[1] *Simpharum*,[2] called *Comphori*, is greatlie lauded for the healing or helpyng of the Carbuncle, beyng ground or beaten betwene twoo stones, and warme applied to the place. So is the herbe cal'ed *Scabios* in the same manner; so is the Lilie rootes rosted and brused and warme laied on. Lette not the greate white onion rosted, and the pith in the middest beyng taken forthe, stopped with good Triacle or *Mythridatum* warme and applied to the place, bee forgotten; for some use none other thinges for the Carbuncle to cure it. Also consider this: to kepe the bodie temperate in eating. Beware of repletion[4] and swetyng: tarte sauces, Limondes, Sorell, Oringes, thinne wine with water is good,[5] but no suger or swete thinges. Forgette not sweete perfumes of Rose water, cloues, maces, vinegar in a perfuming pan, and haue the stomake annointed with oyle of maces, and the complet ointment of Roses, of eche ij scruples, & *Gallœ muschata* x graines, and dip in a linnen cloth in white waxe, oyle of Roses, white and red Saunders, and the powder of orientall Pearles, fine bole Armen, and the swete woodde of Aloes with Rose water made warme in a little vessel vpon charcole and be not without a good Pomcamber made of Storax, Calamite[7] three dragmes, *Laudani* half an vnce, flowers of water Lillies, Violettes, the wood of Aloes, Spikenarde, of eche a dragme and a halfe; the three Saunders, of eche half a dragme; Cinamon two scruples, Mastike xx graines, white Poppie seede, Campher, of eche a Scruple; Amber and Muske, of eche three graines, with rose water, in a warme Morter; make Pomamber, make a hole in it, and putte a silke lace through it, and weare this against corrupted

Side notes: Good note[3] for the Pestilence. Pestilence[6] perfume. Pomeamber against the Pestilence. Cordiall.

---

[1] Ed. 1564, simples. [2] Ed. 1564, Simphatum.
[3] Eds. 1564, 1573, notes.
[4] Ed. 1564 reads, "Beware of repletiō, light Fishe with tarte sauces."
[5] Ed. 1564 omits "is good." [6] Ed. 1564 omits "Pestilence."
[7] Ed. 1573, Calamitie; ed. 1578, Calaniitie.

aire. The bodie must haue benefite by Purgation with Clister, or Suppositer, or some Potion, as the sirup of Roses solutiue three vnces, confection of Hameche fiue dragmes, and water *Purgyng.* of Endiue iiij vnces, mingled together, and drinke it[1] at once in the Mornyng; or *Benedicta laxatiua* with water of Buglosse. Be not without *Manus Christi* to eate often tymes, and the conserue of Roses to eate before meate daiely. Beware of muche slepe, whiche will make the heate double about and within the harte, for slepe draweth in heate, and in tyme of wakyng it is spread abroad, and the heate draweth to the extreames, as handes, heade, and feete. Sir, forget not this, I praie you.

Antonius.

No, maister doctour, I warrant you I haue noted it well; and though it helpe not me, yet I trust it shall doe good to others when I am gone.

Medicus.

Now, sir, I will take my leaue for a time; my calling is suche that I must depart, and diuers of my pacientes diligently[2] doe loke for me, as the birdes dooe for the daie after the[3] colde winters night. And as tyme and occasion shall serue, I will returne. I haue hidden nothing from you that maie be a meanes to your health, for when life is gone, farewell altogether, wife, children, gold, landes, Treasures, and all the golden glorie of this worlde, and frendes also. Therefore, seyng life is the best iewell whiche bringeth delices[4] to the harte, pleasures to the eye and eare, *An Epicures talke.* swete sauors to the sence of smellyng, and many hidden Treasures; knowledge to the vertue of understandyng; what is he that would make suche an exchaunge if it were possible to the contrary? To forsake his golden bedecked bedde,[5] with sweete slepes, to lye vtterly loste, rotten, forgotten and stinkyng, in a filthie pit of darkenesse, inclosed and bewrapped[6] with wormes. As by example we maie see the multitude of graues in euery Church-yarde, and greate heapes of rotten bones, whom ye knowe not of what degree

---

[1] Ed. 1564 omits "it." [2] Ed. 1564, which diligently.
[3] Eds. 1564, 1573, a. [4] Ed. 1564, brings delites.
[5] Eds. 1573, 1578, heade. [6] Ed. 1564, wrapped.

thei were, riche or poore, in their liues. Therefore, sir, to conclude, plucke vp that weake harte, rejoyce, be glad, and caste awaie all care, I warrant you.

Antonius.

Gramercies, maister doctor, I haue put you to pain with muche talke and questions. I will kepe them in memore, thei shall not be forgotten of my part. Euen so forget not your promise in commyng to me again, my trust is in you: we shall make daily exchange, cunnyng for gold, and loue for labor; yours I am. Haue,[1] take you that to buye you a newe Mule, a footeclothe, and a goune.

Medicus.

What meane your mastership? Well, giue me your hande; and here is myne, with myne harte also, euer yours at com- maundmente as your owne. Thus fare you well, vntill my returne; in the meane while passe the tyme with some pleasaunt companie. Eate good broth made of chickens, leane Mutton, roste a little Partriche, eate light leauened breade; beware of grosse meates, Beefe, Porke, &c., and salletes, strong wine, Spice, sweete meates, and rawe fruites. I praie you remember this, and drinke your Diacodion at night to reconcile slepe again, and be somewhat laxatiue.

A nice gentleman.[2]

Diete.[2]

Antonius.

I thanke you moste hartly; fare you well.

Medicus.

Crispine, where are you. Is it not tyme to depart? We haue taried here verie long, but not without gaine.

Crispine.[3]

Or we depart here in this garden, good Master *Tocrub*, sit doune here a little while, and I will write, for I knowe you are a good

---

[1] Ed. 1578, haue. [2] Omitted in Eds. 1573, 1578.
[3] For "Or we depart," &c., ed. 1564 reads:

Crispine.

Sir, I haue thought it a moneth since our commyng hether: you haue been sente for eight tymes this after noone, and twoo of your pacientes are dedde this daie.

Medicus.

That is no maruell, for who can hold that will awaie. I shall haue more penne manne; you were borne in an other lande, and can not well pronounce Englishe, but speake it indiffrent well. I praie you tell me some verie true experte medicens againste the Pestilence, and I will write them, and putte them in my booke at home. And first of two or three sirupes.[1]

Medicus.

Indeede for that you counte me rude in English, marke what I saie in plain Latin. A learned man hath with greate modestie, after long studie, written it, I warrant you. *Ref.*[2] *Syrupus acetositatis citri, ac syrupi de granatis æque, ʒ v; Syrupi de agresta, ʒ iiij; aquarum Buglossæ acetosæ pariter, ʒ i, ſs; misce quo syrupus acetosus cum speciebus triasantalorum temporibus Peslilentiæ diebus sumptus est bonus. Ref.*[3] *Syrupi de pomis descrip. huborregis, ʒ vi; Syrup acetoli de succo acetose equaliter, ʒ iii;*[4] *Syrup. Granatorum, ʒ ii; Aquarum Buglosse*[6] *lupulorum eque, ʒ i, ſs. misce.*

For the hote cholerike Pestilence Rabi Moyses in sui Aphor. Par. xxxi.

In[5] the Melancholike Pestilence.

worke then I can put my hande vnto. It is now a golden worlde with me, and with you also.

Crispinus.

God continue the same. I would thousandes were sicke, but I would haue none dedde but the beggers that doe trouble the world, and haue no money to paie. I praie you what thinke you of maister Antonius; shall he escape it or no?

No winde but it dooth tourne some men to good.

Medicus.

I haue his plentifull rewarde, and money for you also. I haue had lōg talke with hym. But to bee plain with you, I thinke neuer to se hym againe aliue. He was paste cure or I came to hym, and he could not skape; therefore I kepte hym with longe talke, but I spake but softly.

Crispine.

Then I perceiue your talke was vnprofitable to him. Yet I wrote it in a little paper booke in my hande.

Medicus.

Not vnprofitable if the Phisicion come in the beginnyng or augmentyng of the sicknesse. But in the full state of this sickness, it is most dangerous, because death will preuente it or it cometh to the declinacion. Oh, it is a strong poison if the Pestilence crepe to his harte.

Crispine.

This man loued you well in his life, &c. [proceeding as on p. 55, "He loued me," &c.]

[1] Ed. 1578, scrupes.
[2] These recipes are printed as they stand in old ed.
[3] Ed. 1573, *Refe.* [4] Ed. 1573, iiii.
[5] Ed. 1573, For. [6] Ed. 1573, Bugalossae.

Item, one moste excellente in vertue againste the moste sharpest Pestilence and the sore, but it is costly, I warrant thee. *Ref. Endiuæ, Lactucæ Scariola acetosæ, semenis Citri mundati a cortice, singulorum ℥ i; Rosarum Rub. violarum florum, Nenupharis folio, Buglossæ, Borraginis, ana ℥ fs; florum Rosmarini, ℥ iii; Succorum pomarum dulce, santalorum succorum Limonum Citrangulorum, ℥ ana i; Cit, ℥ iii; Garyophillorum, Ciamomi, Ligni aloes, ana, ℥ ii fs. Maceris Croci, ℥ ii fs; Macerenur in aquis Melissæ, Buglossæ, violarum acetose, Boraginis, Rosacii, singulorum, ℥ vi; per triduum et per asembicum in balneo mariæ distillentur cui addatur succharum q. s. et fiat iulep cum acelositate citri q. f. dosis est, ℥ iii.*

These are good with Endiue water for flegm or Bloud.

In the winter putte in Calaminte and Setwall rootes.

Crispine.

Gramercies, good Master Doctor *Tocrub*, I haue written theim; I praie you teache me one or twoo kinde[1] of Pilles.

Medicus.

Ref. Aloes partes duas, Myrrhæ, Croci, aque partem vnam conficiantur pil, testatur Rasis nunquam vidi aliquem deuorantem hanc medicinam qui non liberetur aut perseruaretur ad epidemia.

Three graines of Barlie waight, daily drinke it in a little wine.

Item.

Ref. Aloes selecti, ℥ i; Scabiose, zedoarie, Tormentiliæ, Diptamni ana, ℥ i; Myrrhæ, ℥ fs; Xiloaloes, rosarum rub. Nucis moschate, Charyophilorum, Cinamomi, Santalorum, Spodii de Canna Ana, Ğ xv; Agarici albi leuis, ℥ ii fs; Salis Gemmæ, ℥ fs; cum Syrupo acetositatis citri formentur pil, dosis est, ℥ i.

Ioannes Damascemus. put it in the iuce of three hearbes, as betonie, punpenell and germander.

Crispine.

Teache me a Pomeander, I praie you.

Medicus.

Ref. Florum nenupharis, violarum, rosarum, florum buglossæ,

---

[1] Ed. 1573, kindes.

Santatorum oinm[1] *spodii, ana.* ℈ *i ſs; camphoræ,* ℈ *iii;*   A Pincelle
corticum citri, macis, nucis moscate, maiorani, ozimi, gario- Pomeamber
fillati, charibi, styracis, cal, cardamomi, zediarii, lignialoes, cucubarum,
ana, ℈ *ſs; laudani optimi,* ℈ *iij; ambræ, musci ana,* ℈ *ſs. Conſice pilas parphoratas cum mucilagine dragani; disolue in aqua rosata et foraminibus abscondantur muscus, ambra, et camphora, deinde malexentur. Vel talis mutata a Ioanne Arculano.*

Crispine.

I haue also written this; now of a trim perfume or twoo, and a pouder, and an electuarie, and a cordial ointment against the Pestilence, and then no more.

Medicus.

Ref. Benzoin, ℈ *iii; ligni Aloes,* ℥ *ſs; sacchari candi,* ℥ *i ſs; moschi finissimi,* Ġ *xi; cum muco draganti ex aqua rosata fiant rotule depressæ pro suffitu.*

Vel talis.

Ref. Carbonis salicis, ℥ *iii; cinamomi, gariofilorum, ana,* ℥ *ſs; Styracis, calamite, Laudani, ligni cupressi, benzoini, sachari*   Perfumes
fini, ana, ℥ *iii ſs; rosarum rub. siccarum, florum leuan-* against the Plague.
dule, spicæ ana, ℥ *i; Ambræ musci,* ℈ *i; gummi draganti in aqua rosata dissoluti et cum aqua vitæ q. s. formentur trochisci.*

Item puluis solutiuus.

admirabilis contra Pestem.

Ref. zedoariæ, garriophilorum, zinzeberis, nucis muschatæ, cinamomi, piperis longi, calami aro. baccarum lauri, myrrhæ, aloes, epatici radicum, been Angelicæ, pimpinellæ, agarici, ana, ℥ *ſs; cortice*   A pouder
de radice citri, cardui benedicti, ana, ℈ *ij; camphor,* ℈ *i;* against the Plague.
gentianæ, ℈ *iii; folliculorum sene,* ℥ *ſs; pulcrizentur omnia per se deinde misceantur qui assumatur,* ℈ *i ſs; cum saccharo et aqua betonica.*

Ref. Aquarum rosarum, melisse, oxialidis, ana, ℥ *vi;*   An Epithimum
vini veteris potentis, ℥ *i; aceti,* ℥ *ſs; cortcis citri* against the Plague at the harte.
puluerizati, ℥ *i; rub. spodii, carabe omnium santalorum,*

---

[1] Ed. 1573, *Santalorum omnium.*

ferici combusti, ana, ℈ *i fs; croci*, ℈ *i fs; maceris*, ℈ *i fs; garyophillorum, mucis moschatæ ana*, ℈ *i fs; moschi*, G̈ *v; fiat epithimum pro corde.*

Vel tale.

Rêf. Aquarum Rosarum, Buglossæ, acetosæ, ana, ℥ *iiii; vini Antiqui potentis*, ℥ *ii; boli Armeni Orientatis, subtilissime triti*, ℈ *ii; fiat epithima de quo etiam mane et sero bibere poteris*, ℥ *ii; pro vice.* An Epithemu againste the plage to drink or with scarlet againste the harte.

Electuarium quod aliqui nuncupant salutem populi.

Rêf. Radicum enulæ, ℥ *iii*, ℈ *vi; baccarum Iuniperi, zedoariæ, ana*, ℈ *x; Aristolochiæ rot*, ℥ *ii fs; radicum aristolochiæ longe, zedoariæ foliorum hypericonis, scabiosæ retœi sauinæ, ana*, ℈ *vi; betonice, saluie prassii, spicæ, baccarum lauri, gentianæ, diptamni veri, tormentiullæ, calami aro, ana*, ℥ *fs; adicum assarij, phu, pimpinellæ, seminis ameos, premorsiuæ, corui, macis, angelica, astrucij, santalorum rub. ana*, ℈ *ii; foliorum melissæ, myrrhæ optime, ana,* ℥*fs; castorii,* ℈ *iii; corralorum rubrorum granatæ præp. absinti calementi, zinzebris, piperis nigri, ana*, ℈ *i; caphure*, ℈ *i fs; nucum inglandium nume, xiiii; oxymellis scyllitii*, ℥ *ii; olei terreben*, ℥ *i; mellis dispumati, q. s. fiat electuarium secundum artem qui est minor Decem annorum propinetur*, ℈ *i; qui est ætatis, xv* ℈ *i fs; qui est intra xx.* ℈ *i.; qui est ultra, xx. ii* ℈ *fs.* A noble medicine made by D. Andrewe Galbe of Tridente to the Emperour against the pestilence.

Crispine.

God reward you, good Maister; I praie God of his mercie make the ayre, and our dwellyng places cleane and pleasant, voide of corruption or infection, as by gods grace I will truely make my medicines that I haue written. Lorde, how this gentleman hath loued you well in his life; if he dooe depart this present worlde, will ye not be present at his buriall, Maister doctour?

Medicus.

He loued me as I loued hym, He me for healthe, and I hym for money; And thei whiche are preseruers of the life of manne, ought not to be present at the death or buriall of the same man, therefore I haue taken my leaue, I warrante you, Worldlie freendship

Crispine; I will retourne to hym no more. Thus fare you well till the morowe in the mornyng.

Crispine.

4 I must also depart to my Shop: I haue muche businesse to dooe; I will come to you at your commaundement, maister Doctor. Thus fare you well.

Ciuis.

8 Good wife, the daiely ianglyng and rynging of the belles, the commyng in of the minister to euery house in ministryng the communion, in readyng the Homelie of Death, the diggyng vp of graues, the sparring in of windowes, & the blasyng 12 forth of the blewe crosse, doe make my harte tremble & quake. Alas, what shall I doe to saue my life? ^{The citeezens feare.[1]}

Vxor.

Sir, we are but yonge, and haue but a tyme in this worlde, what 16 doeth it profite vs to gather riches together, and can not enioy theim? Why tary wee here so long? I dooe thinke euery hower a yere vntill we begon; my harte is as cold as a stone, and as heauy as Leade, God helpe me. Seeyng that wee 20 haue sent our children foorthe three weekes past into a good ayre and a sweete countrie, let us followe them. We shall be welcome to your brothers house, I dare say; my sister will reioyce in our commyng, and so will al our freendes there. Let vs take leaue of 24 our neighbours, and retourne merely home again when the Plague is paste, and the Dogge daies ended; and there you maie occupie your stocke, and haue gaine thereof. ^{His wifes counsaile.[2]}

Ciuis.

28 Oh, wife, we knowe not our returne, for the Apostle saieth to you that will saie, To daie or to morowe wee will goe to suche a citie, and buie and sell, and haue gaine, and knowe not what shall happen to morowe. What is our life? It is as a vapour that 32 appeareth for a little tyme, and afterward vanishe awaie; for that ye ought to saie, if the Lorde will and we liue, we will to this or ^{James iii.}

---

[1] Ed. 1564, "The citizen his feare."   [2] Ed. 1564, "his wife her."

that place; and if it please God wee will bothe departe and retourne againe at his good will and pleasure, for wee are in his handes whether so euer wee doe go; and I trust it is not againste Gods commaundemente or pleasure that wee departe from this infected Ayre.

Vxor.

I knowe not what God will in our departyng, But my fleshe trembles when I doe heare the Death bell ryng.

Ciuis.

Yes surely, we haue the Apostle saiyng (for our defence in fliyng), no man euer yet hath hated his own fleshe, but nourisheth[1] and cherisheth it: therefore, who can nourishe his fleshe in a corrupted ayre, but rather doe kill it? Further, I heare[2] a doctour of Phisicke saie that one called Galen, in a booke of Triacle, to one Pison,[3] his friend, that the Pestilence was like a monsterous hungrie beast, deuouryng and eatyng not a fewe, but sometymes whole cities that by resperation or drawyng in their breath do take the poisoned aire. He lauded *Hypocrates*,[4] whiche saieth that to remoue from the infected ayre into a cleaner, thereby, saieth he, thei did not draw in more foule ayre, and this was his onely remedie for the plague: to them that did remaine he commaunded not onelie simple wood to be burned within the Citie of Athens, but also most sweete flowers and spices, perfumes, as gummes and ointementes, to purge the ayre. And, wife, feare of Death enforced many holie men to flie: as Iacob from his cruell brother Esau, Dauid from Saule, Elias from Iesabell. The Christian men from feare of Death did flie the tyrannie of the Papistes, and although these men did not flie the Pestilence, yet thei fledde all for feare of Death; and so will we by Gods grace obserue suche wholesome meanes, and obeye his Diuine prouidence. Also I will leaue my house with my faithefull freendes, and take the keyes of my[5] chestes with me. Where are our horses?

<small>Ephe. v.</small>

<small>Galen ad Pisonem. Non aliter curavi quam aeris mutatione, &c.</small>

<small>Gene. xxii.</small>

---

[1] Ed. 1564, nurished & cherished. [2] Ed. 1564, heard.
[3] Eds. 1573, 1578, Philon. [4] Ed. 1578, Hopocrates.
[5] Ed. 1564, the.

Vxor.

Our thynges are redie; haue you taken your leaue of our[1] neighbours, Man?

Ciuis.

I haue dooen so; now lette vs departe, a Gods blessyng, good wife.

Vxor.

Giue me my horse, Roger.

Roger.

Maistres, he is here ready at your hand, a good geldyng. God bless him and sweete sainct Loye.

Ciuis.

Bryng forthe myne also, and let the seruauntes forget nothyng behinde them, specially the Steele Casket. Let vs ride faire and softely vntill we bee out of the Toune.

Vxor.

How pleasante are these sweete feeldes, garnished with faire plantes and flowers! the birdes doe syng sweetely and pitifullie in the bushes; here are pleasant woodes. Iesus, man, who would be in the citie againe? Not I, for an hundred pound. Oh, helpe me! my horse starteth, and had like to haue been vnsadled; let me sitte faster for fallyng.

Ciuis.

He is a birde eyed iade, I warrant you, and you are no good horsewoman, for I did neuer see you ride before in all my life; but exercise will make you perfecte. Your mother was a good horsewoman, and loued ridyng well as any gentlewoman that euer I knewe in my life. Well, she is gone, and we must followe: this is the worlde.

Vxor.

I neuer was so farre from London in all my life. How farre haue wee ridden alreadie, sir, I praie you?

Ciuis.

Wife, we haue riden x mile this mornyng.

---

[1] Ed. 1564, your.

Vxor.

What toune is this, I praie you, sir?

Ciuis.

This is Barnet, whereas Samuel your soonne was nursed; and yonder is Richarde Higmers house; we will see hym as we doe returne home againe; we will not tary now, because euery Inne is pestered with Londoners and Cariers, and it is earely daies. How like you this toune, dame?

Vxor.

A pretie streate; but me thinke the people go very plain; it is no citie as I do suppose by their maners. What house is this at the tounes ende, compassed with a Moate?

Ciuis.

Here dwelleth a freende of ours; this is called the Folde. And[1] here before is Dansers hill, and Rigge hill.

Vxor.

What greate smoke is in yonder wood? God graunt it be well.

Ciuis.

It is nothyng but makyng of Charcole in that place.

Vxor.

Why, is Charcole made? I had thought all thynges had been made at London, yet I did neuer see no Charcoles made *A wise cockney.* there: by my trouth, I had thought that thei had growen vpon trees, and had not been made.

Ciuis.

You are a wise woman; thei are made of woode. But how like you this Heath? Here was foughten a fearfull feeld, called Palme Sondaie battaile, in kyng Edward the fowerthes time; many thousandes were slain on this grounde; here was slaine the noble Erle of Warwicke.

Roger.

If it please your maistership, my graundfather was also here with twentie tall men of the Parishe where[2] I was borne, and none of

---

[1] The words "And here . . . hill" do not occur in ed. 1564.
[2] Ed. 1564, whereas.

them escaped but my graundfather onely. I had his Bowe in my haund many a tyme; no man can[1] stirre the stryng when it was bent; also his harnesse was worne vpon our S. Georges backe in our churche many a cold winter after; and I heard my Grandame tell how he escaped.

Ciuis.

Tell me, Roger, I praie thee, how he did escape the daunger.

Roger.

Sir, when the battaile was pitched and appointed to bee foughten neare vnto this Windmill, and the Somons giuen by the Harottes of Armes, that Speare, Polaxe, blacke Bill, Bowe and Arrowes should be sette a worke the daie followyng, and that it should bee tried by bloudie weapon, a sodaine feare fell on my Grandfather; and the same night, when it was darke, he stale out of the Erles campe for feare of the kynges displeasure, and hid hym in the Wood; and at length he espied a greate hollowe Oke Tree with armes somewhat greene, and climbed vp partly through cunnyng, for he was a Thatcher, but feare was worthe a Ladder to hym; and then by the helpe of a writhen arme of the Tree he went doune and there remained a good while, and was fedde there by the space of a Monethe with olde Ackornes and Nuttes whiche Squirels had brought in, and also did in his Sallet keepe the Raine water for his drinke, and at length escaped the daunger. [Barnet field, Anno 1471.]

Ciuis.

So he might for anie stripes that he had there; he was well harnessed with a Tree, but I neuer read this in the Chronicle.

Roger.

There be many thinges (and it shall please your Maistership), whiche are not written in the Chronicles, I do think are as true as John your man doe read vnto me when we doe go to bedde, almost euerie night. I shall neuer forget them: fare wel, good Ihon!

Ciuis.

What are they, Roger?

---

[1] Ed. 1573, could.

Roger.

Marie, sir, he tolde me in the olde tyme howe Horses, Sheepe, Hogges, Dogges, Cattes, Rattes, and Mise did speake, and I dooe partlie beleue that, for as muche as our Parate will saie, Parate is a minion, and beware the Catte, and she will call me Roger as plaine as your Maistership; and although Dogges haue loste their speache yet thei doe vnderstande. When I doe whistell Trowle will come; he will fetche my gloue, my bolte in the water, or stoope or lye doune when I bidde hym; and surelie he whiche doeth vnderstand and here what I doe saie maie speake also, but that there are so many languages now adaies he can not tell whiche to speake and to leave all alone, and tourneth all too plaine barkyng as women doe, when as thei doe fall from reasonyng into scoldyng.   *Dogges and women.*

Ciuis.

Thou foolishe knaue, what meanest thou to speake thus? Dogges did neuer speake; thei doe want reason. For there are three thynges to be considered in eche l:uyng creature: the first is vegitable, wherein a man, Dogge, and tree are all one. The second is sensible; in this man and Dogge are all one. The third is, where man excelleth all other creatures, where he hath reason and iudgement, hauynge acte to dooe well and power to doe euill; althrough[2] this reason man doeth speake. The beaste wanteth reason, therefore he speaketh not, &c. But Dogges are taught by custome, and not moued by reason.   *Three things to consider[1] in all creatures.*

Roger.

Well, sir, our Iohns booke shall confounde your talke, for I did see it in writyng; and that whiche is written I will beleue, and follow by Gods grace, and no more.

Ciuis.

Why, will ye doe no more for mee then I haue commanded you by writyng? You are an honest felowe.

---

[1] For "to consider" (the reading of ed. 1578) eds. 1564, 1573, read "considered."

[2] Eds. 1564, 1573, through.

5 ★

Roger.

When I came to you first you gaue me a scroll of parchment, wherein saied you, do no more but as this commaundeth, Rogers writyng. and I will aske no more of thee, but allowe thy seruice. Nowe, in case your Maistership with your horse fell both into the myre ouer the eares, if it were not in my writyng to helpe you bothe forthe I haue doen you no euill seruice. Ha, ha, ha, how cracke you this nutte?

Vxor.

It were a good deede to cracke your pate, you saucie verlet. Gods dentie, Iacke sauce, whence came you?

Roger.

Forsoothe, out of the countree, Maistres nisibicetur, as fine as fippence! How pretely you can call verlet and sweare by Gods dentie! God blesse you, I did neuer see you stomble before.

Vxor.

Out, Roge and Slaue! Auaunte, villaine! Out of my sight, knaue!

Roger.

I thinke you learned your Retorike in the vniuersitie of Bridewell; you were neuer well wormed when you were young.

Vxor.

Sir, you do ride too fast; haue you not heard what this honest man haue saied to mee?

Ciuis.

Dame, all thinges must be taken in good parte; I heard nothing. If any thing bee amisse, at our retourne it shall be amended; we must haue one ridyng foole by the waie, so that it bee dooen merelie and exceade not. Well, felowe, you doe beleue that beastes will speake, because it is written so of them?

Roger.

That I will; if that my Maistres will holde her peace, I will proue it.

A DIALOGVE.

Vxor.

I praie you geue eare to no suche trifles and lies, good houseband.

Ciuis.

I praie you bee contente, it is as good to heare a lye whiche hurteth not as somctyme a true tale that profiteth not. Tell on geently, Roger, a Gods name; ride nere, and let vs be merie.

Roger.

It so chaunsed in the pleasaunt tyme of Maie, a lustie young Lion after his praie or newe eaten spoile did lye him doune to slepe, and yet being a slepe the beastes that were nere hande did quake and tremble in beholding of his most fearefull countenance and fledde awaie. The poore cillie Mouse crept out of her small caue and came softelie, thinkyng no harme, and plaied aboute the Lyon and piped merelie; wherewith the Lyon awaked sodainlie and was angrie, caught the[1] Mouse forthwith, thinkyng to haue deuoured it, but this poore Mouse kneled doune vpon her knees and held up her handes, saying, I haue offended your lordship, I praie you therefore forgeue me and let me haue my life, and once, perhaps,[2] I shall requite it you again;[2] whereat the Lion smiled, and let her passe awaie in peace. Within fewe daies after[2] the same Lyon was taken in a strong Net, thinking neuer to haue been deliuered, and cried most fearfullie with desperation. But gentle Margerie Mouse with her companions[3] withal speede came runnyng, and with sharpe filed teeth did gnawe and shread the strong cordes which intrapped the Lion, wherewith hee stoode at libertie and wente his waie. This is true, when Mise and Lions did speake. I wil abide by the same, sir, if it shal please your Maistership.

The tale of the Lyon.

Pacience in pouertie.

Ciuis.

No, surelye, Lyons nor Mise did neuer speake, Roger, but some wise manne hath written this to this ende, that like as crueltie is to bee vtterlie auoided, euen so ingratitude is *Note this.*

---

[1] Eds. 1564, 1573, this. [2] Omitted in ed. 1564.
[3] The words "with her companions" are not found in ed. 1564.

to be abhored. We maie hereby consider that verie poore menne in the time of trouble maie helpe the mightie and strong,[1] and oftentymes doe indeede. Why should then the greate lorde forget the benefite of a poore grome, which many waies maie pleasure him: (if the simple Mouse wer from the Lyon) then the gentleman were most wretched, in occupation and drudgerie most vile, if poore and simple men in the tyme of extreme persecution by God's prouidence haue deliuered the oppressed, whiche persecuted or oppressed men[2] since are come to greate promotion, both spirituall and temporall, doe forget the same benefites again. It were not only the partes of infidels, but also more ingratefull then beastes, as horses which haue rescued their maisters in battaile, and dogges which would neuer eate after their maisters death, but die upon their graues. Another kind of ingratitude is with Judas, when one bestowe a benefite upon a man, the same manne to inuente to murder his frende. *Knauishe ingratitude.* As if a man in the tyme of colde should finde a snake, and for foolishe pite put hym into his bosome to warme him, I thinke his nature is to sting the man; or if a Shepherde shoulde bryng a young Wolfe vp emong his Lambes and geue him Milke, surelye he would fall to bloode at length and kill the Shepherde himself. *Boner[3] and his fellows.*

Roger.

Sir, you haue well expounded my tale, now I knowe your meaning. I perceiue it is not good keping of such vnkind beastes; they are verie costly and perilous, and would haue Jacke Drakes medicene. *Jacke drake.* Sir, vpon a tyme when quacklyng Duckes did speake and caklyng hennes[4] could talke, whiche indeede are continually[5] companions bicause they are Foules (Marie of sundrie kyndes and names); for Duckes and all water foule doe not onely take the benefite of goodly pondes, riuers, and pleasaunte waters in the time of hotte Summer, with manie deintie meates, and at their pleasures they doo take the commodetie of the lande also. The

---

[1] In the margin of ed. 1564 is written "Ingratitude."
[2] Omitted in ed. 1564.
[3] The marginal annotation in ed. 1564 is 'Marke this.'
[4] Ed. 1564, and Hēhes kackling.   [5] Ed. 1564, continuall.

lande birdes doe but onely liue vppon the lande as footemen; as for Haukes and fleyng birdes of the woodde whiche daielie persecuteth eche other, as murderers doe innocentes or cruell riche men the poore that would liue in reste, I medle not with them. Vpon a time the Drake with the[1] duck and his neighbours, the Gese, beyng pleasauntlie disposed; as Iudas was, in plaiyng the traitour; onely to destroie the lande foules to the ende that they might enioye both land and water together at their pleasure. After the example of couetous men that would haue all thinges in their handes, and when one manne hath[2] anie good profitable trade to liue vppon they will couette or vse the same, although their poore neighbours do perishe, and that is the cause of muche trouble, good maister, now adaies, that euerie callyng doe pinche and poule eche other, and where the hedge is lowest that commonlie is sonest cast to grounde, but the stronge stakes will stande in the storme. (I speake not of the lustie lawiers nor the mighty marchauntes; no, no, I will obserue nothing in them, let euerie Fatte stande vpon his owne bottome.) Nowe, saide the Drake to the lande fowles, good cosins, we are muche bounde vnto you for your daiely entertainement, good chere,[3] and companie;[4] we with our wiues and children are muche bounde vnto you; you are moste naturall unto vs, we daielie feede and take of youre commoditie, come at our pleasures. Nowe, therefore, take parte with vs, and vse your pleasure upon the Water; there is plentie of young Frie, and Fishe greate store, Sallet herbes of sonndrie kyndes, good against euery wound or grief, both meate and medicine, &c. Oh Lord, what pleasure is there to be had! come, sweete hartes, and let us take our progresse to the pleasaunt Riuer of Tagus, whereas the sandes of that flood are precious golde; there is both pleasure and riches; go and gather wealth and treasure; here is pouertie, there is sweetness, and here but stinkyng doung hilles; there is libertie, and here in bondage; there is ioye of the mynd, and here dailey feare of the Fox, that false Traitour. This sweet tale pleased well the lande fowles, as it is often tymes seen that faire woordes make

Traitours.

Rogers obseruation.

Comparisons.

---

[1] Ed. 1564, his.   [2] Eds. 1564, 1573, haue.   [3] Ed. 1564, in good chere.
[4] Ed. 1564, daiely companie.

fooles fain; notwithstandyng, the Cocke saide vnto the Drake: Gossippe, our bringyng vp hath[1] been by lande, and our[2] fathers also; we can not swim, wee haue no webbes in our feete to rowe withall as you have; we feare drownyng. What, saied the Drake, what nedeth these wordes emong frendes? Vse maketh perfitenesse; wee will teache you to swim by arte as well as we doe by nature (nothing is to hard[3] to willing minds). Well, let vs go together; haue with you, saied the Cocke. Then, verie womanlie, the Duck did take the Henne by the hand, following their house- *Marie when freudes doue meete.* bandes, whiche were arme and arme walking before; the Chickens and the Ducklynges followed in a goodlie traine, as it had been to a sumpteous Mariage betwene the Cockes eldest soonne with the pale face and the Drakes doughter with the pretie foote. At the water side the Drake with all the water foules did stoupe lowe and receiue their carriage, and when they were all a cockehorse *Horsemen.* together they wente into the water; and eftsones, when the Drake gaue his watche woorde, the water foules did all sincke at ones, and all the land foules were sodainly in a wrecke, and manie of them perished, and some with muche a doe came to lande, as the Cocke and the Henne, whiche returned home with care and shame, and liued long in lamentation and remained solitarie, without companie of water foules. The Fox, whiche had games a both sides, made the league with a learned oration painted ful of Rhetorike, between them; declaring what vnitie was between brethren and the fruictes of[4] peace, and so reconciled the water foules to lande, where was a feined truce taken with muche dissemblyng yet very good chere, shaking of handes and[5] kissyng, &c. Greate was the feaste at the Cockes place; the Nightyngale was there to pleasure them with Musike, the[6] Cuckowe songe the plaine song soberly, muche daunsyng, and after the same a costlie banket. As you knowe the maner of the water foules dooe commonly sitte nere the grounde, but land foules dooe mounte vp to perche,[7] and so they did. And when

---

[1] Eds. 1564, 1573, haue.   [2] Eds. 1573, 1578, your.
[3] Eds. 1573, 1578, deare.   [4] Ed. 1564, and.   [5] Omitted in ed. 1564.
[6] The words 'the Cuckowe ... soberly' are not found in ed. 1564.
[7] Eds. 1564, 1573, perke.

all were at reste, secretly the cocke sent by the catte a token to the Fox to come and doe execution emong the ingratefull[1] traitors. The cat was glad and ran to the Foxe, findyng him in praier,[2] and shortly declared thambassage; the Fox at the first refused so hainous and 4 bloodye a deede, declaryng his indifferencie and righteousnesse, like a father emong his children,[3] and also what euill opinion manie creatures causelesse had in hym. Marie, saied he, I loue the cocke and his wife verie well; I also know how the water foules haue 8 doen, I haue made the vnitie betwene theim. I will therefore not be seen in this matter my self, but two of my sonnes shal do the feate; goe you[4] before and clime in at the Windowe and open the dore. So in fine it was dooen; sodainlye the water foules paied for 12 the Malte grindyng, and were slaine like flatryng ingratefull villaines. And this is John Drakes medicen: my[5] tale is long.

Ciuis.

This tale is well tolde; Roger, I thanke thee. Ingratefull people 16 and flatterers bee moste wicked, and the children of Judas. If any man be prepharred by another man and made riche, if this riche manne shoulde forget that benefite to his friende if he fell into pouertie, whether would the poore mans lacke more vexe himselfe or 20 the ingratitude of hym that he had pleasured (whiche, perhaps, hath saied, if euer I haue suche a Mariage, yea, or such a ferme, and in case if he be of the clergie, suche a bushoprike, pre- Note this note bendarie, &c., thou shalt not want as long as I can well. 24 helpe; I wil neuer forget your curtesie showed to me in these my daies of trouble)—how saiest thou by this question, Roger?

Roger.

Sir, sauyng your reuerence, you maie cal it ingratitude, but slaun- 28 dering no man, in my iudgement it is plaine knauerie, Knauerie. therefore it is good trying of friendes before need do require; as the man which taught his sonne to kill a swine, and put hym in a sacke

---

[1] Ed. 1564, gratefull.   [2] Ed. 1564, in sacrifice and praier.
[3] The words 'emong his children' are not found in ed. 1564.
[4] Omitted in ed. 1564.
[5] The words 'my tale is long' are not found in ed. 1564.

all bloodie, and secretlie to proue his friendes, whiche of theim would helpe not onelie to hide the slain man, but also helpe to conuaie him in safetie. And to conclude, in the tyme of trouble, emong many be found but one.

A frende at neede.

Ciuis.

Marie, God defende that murder should bee cloked by friendship, whiche, although it be, yet God often himself will take vengeaunce, be it neuer so cloase, as example, in Caine. I like not this example of thyne.

Secret murther openlie punished.

Roger.

I haue better in store, if you will here it.

Ciuis.

Saie on, a Gods name, it is good passing the tyme; but me think we ride to faste: we haue daie enough. How doe you, wife? What chere with you, Susan,[1] mine harte?

Vxor.

Well, sir, I thanke you; I heare your talke well. God be with our frendes at home, and forgeue our foes, and ende these plagues at London, and amend al people that through sinne haue moued God to plague vs.

Ciuis.

It is well saied, good wife. Amen, Amen. Remember your talke, good man Roger.[2]

---

[1] 'Susan, mine harte' omitted in ed. 1564.
[2] Ed. 1564 proceeds as follows:—

Roger.

Sir, in our countree there was a man whiche by occupacion was a Frier (or [of ?] Religion whether you will): I did knowe him well; he wore a graie cote well tucked vnder his corded girdle with a paire of trime white hose. The knaue had a good legge (for his brother was a Yeoman of the Garde, which was a great wrestler): Marie, this Frier although he did rise to the Quere by darcke night, he neded no candell, his nose was so redde and brighte; and although he had but little money in store in his purse, yet his nose and cheekes were well set with currall and rubies; and I doe remember the gentleman had one greate orient pearle in his right iye. He neuer trauelled without Aquaeviti and spectacles and fine Nedles with a quarter staffe in his neck, whiche he called a blesse-beggar. He had

A tale of a Frier.

Roger.

Maister, it giueth me in mine harte that wee[1] shall neuer meete altogether againe in London.[2]

Ciuis.

Wherefore?

many proper colacions and pardons in store; he song his prickesong verie trime; he would have been lothe that any should haue song one note aboue him in the Quere. He was welbeloued in the countree, speciallie emong women; a close man. He was neuer without a bale of dice; Marie, he vsed no foisting nor cogging; he plaied well at tables, and of all meates he moste loued a fat Pigge and a pudding, but he might not awaie to eate Communions nor read the scripture, it euer went against his stomacke, but he was cockhope for Portas matters and cakes. I dare saie he could raise belzebub and bring deuils to crepe and crouche in a circle; also he had the Foolosophers stone and taught many his secretes therein. Upon a tyme this holy Frier in the moneth of June traueiled in his pleasaunt prograce with his boie followyng hym, which was in deede his sisters sonne, one yong Renob by name, a pretie young stripplyng: and as thei had walked from the morning vntill tenne of the clocke, after the Frier had saied our ladie Mattens with a Collect of S. Fraunces his patron, he sat downe vnder a hawthorne tree, to rest with his boie also, & gaue eare to the pleasaunte charme of sweete brides, moche commending the Coko, because she kept so constante her plain song, when the Nightingale did sing the distant [descant]. Oh, saied the boie, this were Paradise, if here were meate and drinke for our reliefe; I would desire no better dwellyng. Yes, saied the Frier, it were better to be a Pope, which is aboue all men, Angelles & deuils; which haue the keyes of heauen gates under his girdle: to whom the kinges of the worlde do seruice. That is past my reche, said the boy; I lacke frendes, age, and learnyng to take that dignitie. Who will finde fault? and if thou wert the Pope, my poore boie, said the Frier, by my preferment, what kindnesse wouldest thou shew to me, beyng so moche thy frend? Sir, said the boie, you should be a Latro Cardinall on my right hand, and be half with me in my kingdome. Remember, saied the Frier, your promise; giue me thy hande, my lad; I promise thee I will make thee Pope. Then he raised sir Sathanas, the patron of Popes, transformed the tree where the boie was into kingly palace, with S. Peters throne, with infinite of the clergie, among whom sate this yong Pope. Forthwith came the Frier in this golden dream; very lowly he kneled and put the Pope in remembraunce who he was and what he had doen, hoping to be gratified. To whom sir Pope said: I knowe thee not, thou lowsie beggar and false Frier; I am discended of kingly parentage, aduaunced by God & learning; awaie with thy blacke cursse, awaie! Forthwith the frier by subtle calculacion withdrewe this delusion of his master the deuil; and the late Pope with his pompe became again the Friers boie, sitting in a Birche tree. To whom the Frier said: Now, you false, vile boie, I knowe what you would haue dooen if you had been Pope. Come doune in the deuilles

The Friers delites.

Yong Renob.

Fur and Latro.

The Popes Patrone.

Pride will haue a fall.

---

[1] Ed. 1564, you.   [2] 'in London' omitted in ed. 1564.

Roger.

Sir, vpon a tyme a nomber of Foxes assembled together at a greate banket, where as was greate plentie of Lambes fleshe, Hennes, &c. In the ende of the feaste this blessed companie, lothe to departe, inquired of old Reinold the daie wherein thei should meete againe to bee merie. I will tell you, saied Reinold,[1] when we shal meete againe; and so trained theim vp to a high mountaine, where as there were manie high wayes deriued into sonderie countries. Fare well, saied he, my little children, and follow your fathers steppes; goe euery one a sondrie waie, for we shall neuer mete againe vntill wee doe meete together in the Skinners shop. Sir, I haue waighed the matter; I warrant you it will proue so. One of late[2] departed, I will not name hym[3] unto

A tale of manie Foxes.

name and carry my wallet. And first, for your knauerie, I will make you a banket of birche. And thus my yong master was serued in this sorte.

Ciuis.

Honours do chaunge maners, yet pride will haue a fall. I dooe remember a poore yong man by fortune was aduanced into promotion, to whom one of his olde fellowes came and spake homelie vnto hym, after the olde fashion, as when they dwelte together. In scorne the riche man answered disdainfully, after this manner:

Take me as I am, not as I was:
We are now no fellowes, it is com to passe.

To whom the other made answere thus againe:

Sometime thou wart, that now thou art not,
And now thou art that that thou werst not,
And what thou shalt be tell thou canst not,
Although a churles hart, liue thou maist not.

A churle incarnate.

Well, well, God sende every ship to a good hauen, and send vs peace and sease this plague, that we maie returne home againe to our old acquaintance; for this weeke I doe remember xx good felowes met together at one banket, my very frendes, Marchauntes and others: you know them well, Roger; towardes yong men & honest, great doers, close and just, wittie, I warrant you, to preuent any prouiso in the lone of monie by moneth or yere; no state or time wil hip them; they can wisely colour the matter, for, Roger, that is an art emong marchauntes not to be reueled. God sende me into their companie again! Notwithstanding, I haue been no great doer in lending forth mony.

Closenesse in Vsurers.

Roger.

Maister, it geueth me, &c.

---

[1] Eds. 1564, 1573, Reinard. [2] So ed. 1564. Eds. 1573, 1578, them.
[3] Omitted in ed. 1564.

you, which is dead and buried; my felowe John once did reade his Epitaphe to mee.

Ciuis.

What was it, I praie thee?

Roger.

No, sir; you will be angrie then.

Ciuis.

Surely I will giue no place to anger to chafe my blood; it is perilous in the pestilent time. For next to the seruyng of Almightie God, and my Christian dutie to my neighbour, I will geue my self onely to mirthe, whiche is the greatest iewll of this world. {What wise men should doe to preserue health.}

Roger.

Sir, thus it was an Epitaph of one that was a greate vsurer, couetous, mercilesse and churlishe, but passyng riche; he knewe no ende of his goodes: it made hym look alofte, and manie louted full lowe at his presence, and thus it was written of hym:—

> *Here lieth Gathrall, that neuer did good,*
> *A gentleman degenerate, yet sprong of good blod:*
> *Mercilesse, an vsurer all the days of his life,*
> *An oppresser of poore men, a mouer of strife;*
> *A papiste of religion, a soldiour of Rome,*
> *Here dwelleth his carkas till the daie of dome;*
> *Depriued of riches, spoyled of fame;*
> *Nothyng left in memorie but an euill name:*
> *His iudgement we commende to the seate diuine;*
> *Yet liued*[1] *like a Wolfe, and died like a swine.*

{An Epitaph of a couetous man.}

Ciuis.

Who was this made vpon, Roger? I praie thee tell me.

Roger.

No, so God helpe mee, I will not name hym; inquire it out. But I heard a frende of myne saie that hee had written a booke against Extorcioners and vsurers; whiche if thei amende not he will name them, and paint them forthe, not only them, but their parentes whiche are dead, whiche vsed that vile trade of Vsurie, {Name no bodie.}

---

[1] Ed. 1564, he liued.

procuryng Gods vengeaunce in castyng the pestilence vpon cities, tounes, and countries; causyng pouertie, breakyng vp houses moste aunciente, sellyng to lende vpon gaine, *The fruictes of Vsurie and Extortion.* destroying hospitalitie with infinite incombraunces, by forfiture,[1] statutes, &c. Oh that the Vsurers gooddes were confiscated after their deathes to the common poore, as in case they had slaine themselues, and that thei had no power in lawe to bee will vnto their children that which was gotten in seruyng the Deuill, whiche woulde not prosper to the thirde[2] heire; for euill gotten goodes are euill spent, saied our curate vpon Sondaie. Oh that their[3] *God graunt.* burying were tourned into open castyng forthe emong deade Cattell, and not nombered in the Christian felloweship after death, whiche in life hath been so wicked; so saied our Curate. Sir, you heard not how a manne of late let forthe his cowe by the quarter and by the yere?

Ciuis.

No; I praie thee tell me.

Roger.

There was a manne of late, whiche had one hundreth pounde, whiche he called his Cowe, and secretly did lende her foorthe sometyme by the weeke, and his price was tenne shillynges the weeke; and when her milke became dearer, and many fastyng daies at hande, he called for his Cowe, and saied that she gaue indifferent Milke. But, saied he, I muste put her into a better Pasture, and she shall giue more milke by fiue shillynges in the weeke, &c. And at lengthe white Meate became a little *Of the Vsurers cowe.* *Many Vsurers.* better cheape because of the greate plentie of suche kine in the toune, that his Cowe was broughte home againe because that she was letten so deare. Nowe, because she had dooen hym good seruice, and he had no more but her at home, and calfe he had none by her to kepe vp the stocke. His seruante loued Milke well, and could get none of that Cowe; when his master was from home stale the cowe and ranne his waie, and hetherto hath not been founde neither cowe nor man, and all the milke is gone. Farewell Frost![4]

---

[1] Ed. 1564, forfitures. [2] Ed. 1564, iij. [3] Ed. 1564, the.
[4] The words 'Farewell Frost!' are not found in ed. 1564.

Ciuis.

A merueilous thyng, good Lord! What would suche Grasiers doe if thei had many cattell or kine in store?

Roger. 4

Thei would destroie all the[1] Commonwealth; but we see what mischief thei haue dooen. And[2] also, maister, what a worlde is this? How is it chaunged! it is marueilous, it is monstrous! I heare saie there is a yong woman, borne in the toune of Harborough, one Booker, a Butchers doughter, whiche of late, God wote, is brought to bed of a cat, or haue deliured a catte; or, if you will, she is the mother of a catt. Oh God! how is nature repugnant to her self, That a woman should bryng forthe a verie catte or a very Dogge, &c., wantyng nothyng, neither hauyng more then other Dogges or Cattes haue! Takyng nothyng of the mother but onely as I gesse her Cattishe condition. 8 12

The maide and the catte.

Ciuis. 16

It is a lie, Roger, beleue it not; it was but a Catte: it had Baken founde in the bealie, and a strawe. It was an old Catte, and she a yong Quene; it was a pleasaunt practise of papistrie to bring the people to newe wonders. If it had been a monster, then it should haue had somewhat more or els lesse; But an other Catte was flaied in the same sorte, and in all poinctes like, or, as it were, the self same; thus can drabbes do somtime when thei haue murthered their owne bastardes, with the helpe of an olde Witch bryng a Catte in place. A toye to mocke an Ape withall. Roger, it should haue been a kitlyng first, and so growne to a Catt; but it was a Catte at the first. 20 24

A dogges tricke.

Roger. 28

Yet there are many one do beleue it was a monster; it maie be as your masship saie, for I remember, God a mercie on al cursed soules, as my brother, James Penyngton the Poticarie in Wodstrete

---

[1] Ed. 1564, a.
[2] This passage, from *And also, maister,* &c. to *I praie God that we meete* &c. (p. 79), is not found in ed. 1564.

told me, vppon a time in London when he was a trim young man, of a woman that plaied a pretie Dog tricke, and this was the matter: She kept an Alehouse, she was leane, yellow <small>James tale.</small>
4 skinned, rustie teeth, thinne lipped, staryng eyen, and sometime her face chaunged into palenesse; she seldome laughed but at her neighbours hurt. Her stomacke was full of choler, ergo a pacient, quiet woman; she receiued both roges and harlottes <small>A quiet woman.</small>
8 into her celler; she had very good nappie ale. Mary, of all menne in the parishe she loued not the Conestable, he deseased often tymes her gestes, of verie kindenesse. She inuented a good tourne for masse Conestable, by the practise of a false drabbe; she with the
12 helpe of a pillowe fained to be with childe, and made this shewe to the people, and vsed her accustomed trickes with her gestes in the dead time of the nyght, at whiche time came the Conestable, whom she in her owne persone resisted; so betwene the Conestable and
16 this sober woman, the doore fell doune upon her, whiche willyngly receiued with an hellishe crie, like a wilde Catt yellyng, crying out that she and that she was withall were bothe caste awaie; and so with speede she sent for her owne midwife, and suche like the
20 constables frendes; and so she saied she was deliured of as goodlie a boye as euer a poore woman groned for. His braine pan, &c., was broken; he was christened in the birth, saied thei; his name was Ihon or Ione; he was put in a little coffine. He had a little corner
24 of a Dirige, with Masse of Requiem; the ale wife gaue some Ale pence to praie for his soule; he was buried by his graundame at the steeples ende. The mother all in white attire was brought to bedde. Oh howe she cried, my boye! my sweete boye! man, you had neuer
28 a childe so like you! Oh, cursed knaue Robinson, our Conestable! Oh, murderyng villaine! This good woman (saied she) did see him, but that the bowelles and braines were putrified, that it was no mans sight, the savour was suche. By God, saied the honest
32 woman, it is no lye; were it not for the feare of God, saied her husbande, I would thruste my dagger into him. A greate rumour rose; all men and women wondered vpon Robinson; the father and mother attempted lawe. Robinson had nothyng to defende hym
36 but his office, yet he secretlie offered money to the good manne; and

that made the good wife bold, loking for a greater reuengemente
against the Conestable. The women were sworne before masse
comisarie that it was a boye, and howe the constable did kill it.
Yea, quod masse Comisarie, the gallowes stretche hym: by saincte
Thomas, the Crouner shall knowe of this; so he did. Whereat
Totnam was tourned into Frenche, and all ranne a repungnante
course backe againe againste the ale wife with a quartile aspect.
Then the Graue was opened, the little Coffine opened, and the
Crouner presented with a cat: a goodlie childe. A pretie practise!
Many such Dog trickes are vsed. Ah, ah, ah, my harte! oh the
craftie hores; a Pestilence on them all! This was true, quod Iames.

Ciuis.

Well said, Roger; this is no lie, I assure thee.

Vxor.

Why, man, what should we talke of such matters or of monsters? I thinke there wer neuer none borne of women. Mary, of
swine, kine or sheepe, I haue hard, and once I did see a chicken with
three feete by Goddes deintie, and an other time I did see a pretie
childe whiche looked a squint and had two sightes in the left eye
perde.

Roger.

Tushe, that is no marueile, that maie be by a thyng called impression or some secrete affection of nature; thei saie that one Plinie
and Lycosthenes doe write vppon many suche thynges, and I heard
one saie that a noble woman brought forthe a black childe like a
man childe of the blacke Moores. Her housebande and she were
white, so were all theim in her house; yea, there was not one blacke
Moore in all that land. The marueill was greate; but in fine, a
learned Manne in Physicke founde forthe the cause, that in the tyme
of conception this woman behelde a picture in a clothe vppon the
wall like a More. And so did Jacob vse a meanes with spotted
stickes and water to haue the shepe of spotted colours for his owne
gaine, deceuing Laban: so, good maistres, this blinkyng Gene. xxx.
boyes mother mighte behold an Image double eyed, or els a fearfull

father begotte it that durste not abide by the reckenyng, castyng his
eye to the doore with greate feare.

Ciuis.

4   Well, Roger, well, will you not leave your Rye?

Roger.

Why, sir, we do ride through a Rie field; it maketh me to
remember some Rye.

8   *Vxor.*

Good husbande, I praie you tell me, was there euer any monsters
borne of women? did you euer read of them, good man? tell me.

Ciuis.

12 Yes, forsoothe, good Susan, it is truth; there haue been many
Monsters borne that is an extraordanarie or marueilous in their
shapes, fearefull to behold and wonderous; and marke this, Susan,
when these doe come, euer commeth either the alteration of king-
16 domes, destruction of Princes, greate battaile, insurrection, yearth-
quakes, honger or Pestilence after them.

Vxor.

I praie you tell me some of them.

20   *Ciuis.*

A little before the bloudie battaile between Marcellus and Han-
nibal was a childe borne with a hedde like a Elephant. Anno mundi, 125.
In Armenia twoo children borne, the one without eyen   Anno ante
24 and nose, the other without handes and feete: after   Christum, 141.
these monsters it rained stones in that region.

When the temple of Juno was builded, in the time of Quintus
Tullus, a man childe was borne with twoo heddes, and a maiden
28 childe with all her teeth: this yeere did three Sunnes   163.
appere in the firmament together.   In Rome a childe borne with
fower handes and fower feete; greate Pestilence and famine did
folowe.

Marcus Tullius Cicero being borne the iii daie of Januarii, many Monsters borne and the greate battaile fought betwene the Romans and the Cibrians, about that tyme. What shall I saie, wife? but tyme will not serue: I might since the tyme of Christes Incarnation vntill this daie rehearse many strange monsters, bothe in Asia and Affricke. But specially in Europe, bothe Germanie, Fraunce, Spaine, Englande, Scotlande, &c., twoo or three heddes of one body, many handes & legges to one body, somtyme twoo bodies to one hedde, &c.; the like maner of monsters of beastes, some half hogge and halfe sheepe, some a hogge with the hedde like a man, &c.; so in foules and fishes; moste fearfull to beholde, and still after theim doe come greate battailes, Pestilence, yearthquake, hunger, and marueilous changes in commonwealthes. I haue doen of suche talke of Monsters, Susan.

Ante Christum, 103.

Roger.

In good faithe it is tyme, and please your mastership.[1] I thinke the conditions of men and women now adaies be as monsterous as euer thei were in bodies mishapen. Bad is the best, the worlde amendes like sower ale in Sommer, more worke for Lawiers, more; now is their haruest greate, thei are the workemen, and of very charitie many plaine plowe men, grasiars, and menne of meane callyng put to their helping handes and put their children to this haruest, and all to quiet the people; that I doe thinke in a while there shall be as many of them as there are Parishe Churches in Englande. And loke what the honest curate will quiet in his Sermon in the fore noone; I thinke thei will marre all in the after noone, and bryng matters with coste into Westminster haull; that with Godes worde onely, neither spendyng labour or a penie, might haue been saued at home. These lawiers, I saie, are cunnyng Carde plaiers; thei knowe howe to make their games; thei see what is in other mens handes, thei see the riche deedes of landes, thei peruse the euidences, thei discomforte often tymes their clientes, and for trifles buy the titles; wise men, honest men, men of good conscience, robbing bothe the widowe and father-

Plaine mens charitie.

Carde plaiers.

---

[1] Ed. 1573, masship.

lesse! Thei haue lawe for the matter. It is a bare pasture *Abusers of lawe.*
that thei can not feede on. Thei wil sette all men together by the
eares for the value of a strawe; marke it well what good neighbours
4 thei are, and howe madde thei are in many cases that set them a
woorke. Fellowes are so braine sicke now adaies if thei haue but
tenne shillynges, yea, though thei doe borowe it, will be twoo or
three times a yere at Westminster haule; let wife or children begge;
8 in the ende thei go home many miles, by foolam crosse, by weepyng
cross, by beggers Barne, and by knaues Acre, &c. This *Home againe,*
commeth of their lawing; then thei crie, might doe ouer- *home againe, the market is*
come right, would I had knowen as muche before, I am *doen.*
12 vndoen, &c. For these good workes of the lawyers, Christe saie,
with a blessyng vnto them (after that he had blessed the Scribes,
whiche I thinke were then as our menne and Proctors be at this
daie), wo be to you lawyers, &c., whiche I thinke is, a *A blessyng for*
16 vengaunce or curse be vnto all lawiers spirituall or tem- *euill lawiers.*
porall that doe wrong for bribes, friendship, malice, lande or money,
against the truthe, againste the innocentes, &c. Now, what doe
Lawiers in this pitifull cases, when Gods worde do rebuke them?
20 repent them? No, no; what then? Then thei go about to stop the
Preachers mouthes, or accusyng theim of railyng, slaunderyng, or
sedicion. Rede the ende of the xi chap of Sainct Lukes *Luke xi.*
Gospell: thei vsed Christe so; I tell your masshippe, Light and
24 darkenes can not agree, neither the lawiers and the diuines, untill a
better reformation be had. All this I hearde a wise man saie, and
an honest man too. He said also, nowadaies how mens Fermes are
taken ouer their hedde ten yeres, or their leases are *Note this well.*
28 expired, and how iiij seruyng mens wages for one yere will not paie
for one paire of their hose; And how every poore mans wife will be
as trim as a gentlewoman; she will laie hir self to gage for gaie geare
els. I thinke the daie of Dome is at hande. Euery man in a maner
32 is fallen into loue with hymselfe, either of his proper persone or
apparell; his quallicomes dooe please hym well, or els when he doe
heare hymself with his retricall trications, how he can compounde
the matter. Oh Lorde, it is a sportation to heare the cloutyng
36 beetles to rowle in their ropripe termes: the worlde, and please your

masship, and my maistres honestie and surreuerence of mine owne manhoode, is full of verletrie; no, no, full of knauerie and harlottrie, coueteousnesse; naie, naie, open extortion. Loue, loue? naie, by Ladie, lecherie; Clenlinesse? fie, fie, it is pride. What, I saie? good chere! Tush, tush, starke drunkennesse. Ease, ease? verie idlenesse. Sadde, sober countenance? mark it well: crewell, frounyng, cankered mynded. Pitifull? no, no, spitefull. Euery churle would possesse al alone, and euery lecherer would peruse the faire women hym selfe alone, and so forthe. Marke the worlde, note it well, not onely emong the temporall, but I praie you what see you in the Churche? No spite, no venerie, no coueteousnesse, &c.? Maister, maister, the worlde doe runne a wheeles. Oh, this geare is monsterous and vile. I doe see our Inne; we shall haue good chere; I am glad of that, by Sainct Lambart. I praie God that we meete with some good merie companie after this sadde talke.

Ciuis.

[1]It is time to baite our horses in this toune. If there be any good meate, wee will dine; prepare, Roger, for we haue far to ride this night. Knowe what companie is in the Inne, and whether the house be infected or no.

Roger.

Sir, I was in the haule and there sitteth our hoste, a pleasant, merie man and a good companion, I warraunt hym. I see by his nose that of al potage he loueth good Ale; *Of geastes in the Inn.* he is mounsire graundpanche; he hath chafed the Parsone wonderously, whiche with a paire of spectacles plaith at Tables with hym; he stealeth faste the Table men from him. Our hostes hath a sharpe Nose, thinne lipped, a proper yonge woman with a shrill voyce like a Catte; but when she is pleased I warrante her to be a pleasaunte woman, and full of meritrix. The good man of this *Meritrix.* house bringeth vp youth verie well, and is verie louyng to his sonne; and I perciue he will beare much with hym.

Ciuis.

Wherein?

[1] Here ed. 1564 begins again.

80   A DIALOGVE.

Roger.[1]

When I came into the haull my yonge maister leaned vpon his fathers shoulder with his cappe vpon his hed, spittyng[2] A yonge man
4 and coughyng like a lought.   well brought vp.

Ciuis.

Call the Chamberlaine and let vs haue a chamber seuerally to[3] our selues.[4]
8   *Roger.*

With all spede a Gods name. Chamberlaine, prepare your chamber with all thinges accordingly in the same for my master and maistres. Whip, maister Ostler! with a caste of legerdemaine
12 bestirre you, sirrha, and make a xij[d] of three bottles of The honestie of
stinkyng Haie and a pecke of Oates. You can make a   an hostler.
stoned horse a geldyng, and a longe taile a courtall. You knowe my meanyng well enough; hem, sirrha, I saie nothing but mum. I
16 haue seen you often in Smithfielde.

Vxor.

What, sir sauce? you take vppon you to plaie the Comptroller? goe quietly aboute your owne busines and let the ostler alone.

20   *Roger.*[5]

Maistres, it is merie when knaues are mette. I did see him ones aske blessyng to xii. Godfathers at ones.

Ciuis.[6]

24 This is a comely parlour, very netly and trimely apparrelled, London like; the windowes are well glased, & faire   A Parlour.
clothes[7] with many wise saiynges painted vpon them.

Vxor.

28 I praie you, housbande, what is that writyng in those golden letters?

---

[1] Ed. 1564, Vxor.   [2] Ed. 1564, sittyng.
[3] Ed. 1573, by.   [4] The words 'to our selues' are not in ed. 1564.
[5] This speech of Roger is omitted in eds. 1573 and 1578.
[6] Eds. 1573 and 1578, Roger.
[7] Ed. 1564, "faire clothes with pleasaunte borders aboute the same, with," &c.

Ciuis.

Melius est claudus in via quam cursor preter viam. That is, better is an haltyng man whiche kepeth the right waie than the swift runner, besides, that wandereth a straie.

Vxor.

What is that, man, I praie you?

Ciuis.

Non hominis consuetudinem sed dei veritatem sequi oportet: which is, It behoueth vs not to followe the constitutions or customes of men, but to followe the truthe of Godes woorde. And also there is a good saiyng followyng the same. *The truthe must bee followed.*

Doctrinis variis et péregrinis ne circumferamini. That is, be not ledde or caried about with diuerse or straunge doctrine. Here is more folowyng written vpon the chimney, good wife, whiche I will kepe in store. Oh God, what serpentes thei are, lorde defende me from them! I will rede it to my self. *O mulier omne facinus ausa est plus quam omne, verum nihil est peius nec erit vnquam muliere[1] inter hominum calamitatis.* *The best doctrin is godes Woorde.*

Vxor.

Well man, well; truth seketh no corners; I perceiue there is some noughtie matter that I knowe not, but by one thyng that I doe here you rede, make me thinke all the rest is not well, because the firste worde is starke nought, & that is *O Mulier*, which I am sure is nor neuer[2] was good. I pray you, husbande, what picture is that followyng? *Mulier is a naughtie woorde, saied the gentlewoman.*

Ciuis.

Oh, wife, it was the picture or Effigium of a noble man, whiche in his daies serued a greate[3] noble Kyng, and was like the cutter doune of Trees by the grounde. But if God had not vpon some secrete purpose preuented his labour in the woodde of Antichriste, he would haue vtterly eradicated vp all Papistrie, whiche *The Lorde Crumwell.*

---

[1] Old eds., mulierae. [2] Ed. 1564, euer.
[3] Ed. 1564, moste.

daiely spryngeth out in euery corner, to the hurte of better fruites; but by Godes grace thei shall be confounded, as God wil: but[1] thei spring a pace.

Vxor.

What picture is that whiche hath a gray hore hed, a long goune, and a locke of Gold linkyng his lippes together, with manie goodlie bookes before hym, and a paire of blinde spectacles vpon his nose, with a golden penne fallen from his handes? *This picture synifieth a[2] great clerke euill occupied in kepyng silence.*

Ciuis.

Oh wife, wife, it is a candell couered with a Bushell, and the noble Tallente of wisedome hidden, whiche muste make greate accomptes for kepyng silence.

Vxor.

Sir, in that table enuironed rounde with antikes of sondrie portratures—the ground thereof is hoping Russet—are three pictures, blacke, scholer like, or in mornyng clothyng; the firste of them with a Rake in his hande with teeth of golde, doe stoupe verie lowe, groping belike in the Lake after some thyng that he would finde; and out of this deepe water, aboue the Rake, a little steple. The seconde gapeth vp towardes the Heauen, holdyng the lappe of his Goune abrode, as though he would catche something; and towardes the same lappe or spred goune doth fall as it were a churche with a stiple, and quere, &c. The third man standeth in poore apparell, with a booke in his righte hande, and his lefte hande vppon his breast, with a lamentable countenaunce, in simple apparell. What meaneth this, housbande? *The golden rake. A gaper. A catcher. A poore man.*

Ciuis.

Dame, I dare saie but little to this matter to others, but to you I will speake a little, and not so much as I doe thinke. The first man is one that hath but a verie small learnyng, lesser wit, & lesse honesty. He hath no vertue to prefer him to a[3] liuyng, but onely the name and title of a priest or minister. *I meane no honest or lerned man.*

---

[1] The words 'but thei spring a pace' are not in ed. 1564.
[2] Eds. 1564, 1573, great clerkes. [3] Eds. 1573, 1578, 'a' omitted.

He would faine haue a benefice or personage of some pretie donatiue, he cannot get it at the bishoppes handes : he lacketh Goddes plough. This felowe raketh with the Deuils golden rake, euen in the conscience of the coueitous patrons or conpounders hart, whiche geueth the benefice; he plaieth *Symon Magus*, he will buy it, and with *Judas* the other will sell it, and at length it is gotten for gold, and spent with wickednesse to the slaunder of the Church. God defend us from such rakers and Simoniakers.[1] The second is sicke of the mother, and like vnto heires, when as the fathers haue left theim faire landes, they mourne of the chine, and are never contented, but wimper and whine vntill the mothers are dead; and when it so cometh to passe, their wicked couetousnes by one meanes or other cometh to shame and pouertie. This honest man gapeth for a vouson of a benefice before it is fallen, and doeth catche it or it cometh to the grounde, before the death of the discombent. He will not suffer it to fall into relappe. This man is a steward to a greate man, or kepeth his hall garden or barnes, or is a wise man and a good husband. Looke where his maister is patron ; there he hopeth to be person. He gathereth for his yong maisters, his patrons sonne[s]; his patron must be his executor or some of his maisters kinsmen. This fellow walloweth in benefices, as the Hedgehog doeth with apples upon his prickes, & hath the benefite but of the apple in his mouth ; he getteth nothyng of his promocions but onely one little benefice, yet his master wil snatch at that, either to saue the woll or lambe. And so hee hath onely the shels or glorious titles of promotion, but the geuer hath the swete kernels. God amend this, good wife! The third is one whiche sheweth the state of learned men labouring long time in studie and diuine vertue, whiche are wrapped in pouertie, wantyng the golden Rake or gapyng mouth. This man hath verie fewe to preferre hym to that promotion; he smiteth himselfe vpon the breast, he wepeth and lamenteth that vice should thus be exalted, ignoraunce rewarded with glorie, coueteous men spoilyng the Churche by the names of Patrones and geuers, whiche are Extorcioners and Tellers; they care

Magus and Judas.

Children sick of the mother: remedie is the gallows.

Patrons charitie

Spirituall promotion.

Symonie.

---
[1] Ed. 1564, Simoniakes.

not to whom so that it be raked with the golden racke.[1] Wel, wel, God of his mercie amend this euill Market.

Vxor.

4 Upon that wall is painted a mans skin, and tanned, coloured like vnto Leather, with the skin of the handes and feete, *A Judges skinne.* nayles and heare remainyng; and the skinne is spread abroad, in the whiche is written certaine wordes, which I doe not vnderstand.

8 *Ciuis.*

Wife, I wishe more suche leather or els fewer suche Carcases as suche skinne[2] hath conteined in it. It is the Skin of a wicked Judge, a Lawier, whiche plaied on bothe handes. This *A wicked Judge, his rewarde.* 12 gentleman loued golde aboue God, and crueltie aboue justice; bothe his eares were stopped, his eyen open; hee had respect of persones, specially who brought in lucre, and made hym humble courtesies: them he would defend, although their causes, 16 in righteousnes deserued it not. The innocent he oppressed that wanted, and vndid manie a manne. His maister beyng *A good Prince.* a greate prince (in the whole multitude of the people, and speeciallye of the Lawiers to teache[3] them to decline from euill and *Money doeth greate mischief in the worlde.* 20 do good; to haue the eares open, to heare bothe riche and poore alike in the seate of Judgemente, to haue lame handes in takyng of money, which is the roote of all euil emong them), commaunded his Skin to be flaine from his fleshe, he 24 beyng yet leuyng, roaryng, with blood runnyng from his bodie, and died in a case moste miserable. Uppon whose Skin is this writyng, hangyng in the judgement Halle before the place of Justice:

Judex qui non querit[4] veritatem debet excoriari: A Judge which 28 will (for lucre) not seeke out the truthe (in the lawe) ought to haue his Skin flaine from his bodie.

Vxor.

Here standeth a woman of moste excellent forme in shape, and 32 fairenes in beautie, with a croune of riche golde, with seuen precious

---

[1] The words 'with the golden racke' are not in ed. 1564.
[2] Ed. 1564, leather.
[3] Ed. 1564, 'to certifie them. And to decline,' &c. [4] Ed. 1564, queret.

stones fixed in the border of her croune, couered with a costely mantell from her pappes dounwarde, her breastes naked; the right brest geueth milke vnto the mouth of the yong childe on the right side, and from the left brest floweth blood into the mouth of an other childe: what meaneth this?

Ciuis.

It is a goodly picture, and signifieth the estate of an vniuersitie, or multitude of scholers which cometh to be nourished in learnyng; whiche mother, the vniuersitie, beyng crouned with the seuin liberall artes fixed in her croune; and as manie as tast of her doctrine in the better part in vertue to this ende to doe well, be blessed: thei do tast upon the right breast; but the lefte breaste yeldeth forthe doctrine of Errours, Magiques, Papistrie, &c. To this ende to persecute, robbe, and spoile Christes Churche, God graunt that both these breastes maye geue good milke to nourishe the people of God in one holy doctrine, to eche vocation, to agree in vnitie like brethren, and that the uniuersities maie teache the learned actes and one true religion in this Christ our Lorde.

Vxor.

What is that picture whiche graffeth a golden Impe upon a Leaden stocke, with a bagge of money of greate bignesse hangyng about his necke.

Ciuis.

It should seeme to be a pitifull case; it is a noble, couetous Senior, whiche for goldes sake dooe make disperigiment of his blood, mariyng and sellyng his sonne and heire vnto some Extorcioner, or shamelesse vsurers daughter, whose fruites are so infected on the mothers side that they will become as counterfect, craftie, compounded mettal, and neuer come to the true touch stone againe[1] as pure gold, But corupted through couet- ousnesse and naturall coniunction, as we doe se graffes of trees fixe yonge impes, although the impe be of a fine Pippin, and graffed into an euill stocke. You shal know

[marginal notes: Uniuersitie and fruictes thereof. One pure well geueth but cleane water. Note also that vertue & gentlenesse maketh gentlemen. Euen so auncient blood, wrapped in vice, is but grosse gentlenesse.]

---

[1] Ed. 1564 omits 'as pure gold,' and proceeds 'The fine mettal is so corrupted.'

that fruicte by the tree, a plague prepared for gentlemen for their abuse, and[1] also for poore men matchyng the vngentle gentle.

Vxor.

Upon that Table before you is painted a naked manne, liyng doune wounded, Upon whome feedeth manie Flies with full bellies; and there commeth an other man with[2] a greene braunche of Rosemarie, and[3] beate them awaie.

Ciuis.

It should appeare by the circumstaunce that it is not hurtfull to keepe officers still in place; for when thei haue filled their purses, and haue all thinges accordinglie, they are well; and if thei be remoued eftesones, the newe hongrie Flies will vexe the bodie of the common weath, and neuer cease untill thei be also satisfied, &c.

<small>A Metaphor. The hongrie Flie will fill his beallie.</small>

Vxor.

Yet what is that man, I praie you, that sitteth in a riche throne a sleepe, and one dooe blowe in his eare with a paire of Golden bellowes, and another do picke his purse?

Ciuis.

That same is a mightie persone, ouercome with adulation or flatterie, carelesse swimming in pleasure and vain glory, whom his men do vse like an honie combe, and daiely spoile him of his riches by sondrie fraudes, whiche he perceiueth not.

<small>Flatterie of noble menne.</small>

Vxor.

And what meaneth yonder Mule, holdyng his hed so lowe, with a plaine blacke foote clothe, shodde with golden shoes?

Ciuis.

Wife, silence nowe is beste; I will saie nothyng to the matter. The Mule carieth a Maister that will dooe nothyng but for golde, and the fooles of the worlde that loue debate and strief must shooe this Mule.

<small>Who shall shoe the mule?</small>

---

[1] The words 'and also ... gentle' are omitted in ed. 1564.
[2] Ed. 1564, which with.   [3] Omitted in ed. 1564.

Vxor.

Here is a rowe of pictures like Prelates, painted one by an other in the border, in three partes. The first are barefooted men, barehedded, long garmentes, and bookes in their handes: some of theym are bloodie. The seconde companie are mitred, and shode with Sheperds hookes in one hande, and bookes in the other hande. The thirde sorte haue Swordes in their handes, crouned with triple crounes, clothed in kynglie robes, with frounyng faces, and bookes vnder their feete; and next after them sitteth an olde mangie slaue naked, with a triple Croune, makyng or patchyng of a Nette, from whom goeth as it were menne laden with tounes, woddes, and treasure. *The description of the Romishe churche.*

Ciuis.

Wife, this is the true Churche of God, and the malignaunte Sinagoge of Antichrist figured; firste the true preachers and Martyres of Gods Church, simple menne, whiche folowed most nere the Testament of Christe. After this persecution then entered Confessours, good men which liued well, and accordyng to the Apostles doctrine were good Shepherdes, withstoode the Wolues of heresies, &c.; kept hospitalitie, and liue[d] accordynglie, and wexe[1] as Lambes and good Wheate. Then for the sinnes of Princes and wickednes of men, came in Wolues emong Lambes, Darnell choked the Lordes field, oppressours of Princes, emptiers of Purgatorie, and fillers of helle, raisers of debate, shedders of bloodde, makers of Martyres, menne of warre, destrowers of the true churche, erectours[2] of Idolles, vsurpers of kyngdomes, and treaders of Goddes truthe vnder their vile feete; whiche feete kynges haue kissed, suche is the pride of the Pope. *The description of the prelates of the Romish Churche.* *The Popes Sickenes.*

Then the Pope sitteth all naked, woorkyng nowe through Gods woorde; Antichrist is reueled and seen what hee is, foule, lothlie, clothed in shamefull decrees, wicked lawes and filthie life, and[3] despised of manie nations, saue of his owne children; nowe patched his olde Bottelles, whiche will kepe no new wine, neither can he well peece Christes pure cloth and his ragged *The Popes practice.*

---

[1] Ed. 1578, waxe.   [2] Eds. 1573, 1578, exectours.
[3] Ed. 1564, and is.

tradicions together; neither wil this[1] net pleasure the Churche, in whiche nette hee hath[2] taken the seruauntes of Christe: shed their bloodde. He maie bee rather called a murderer then a fisher; he neuer had sainct Peters nette since the Pope came to the church of Rome; now cloueth he a nette with his rotten Decrees, Counsailes, glosing it with Gods worde. Like the Angell of darkenesse transformed into the similitude of an Angell of light; but his nakednesse is seen for all his title of his holines and riche Croune. Now as manie as will not obeie his maistership, he geueth awaie their kingdomes, dukedomes, prouinces, and gooddes, after the example of his patrone, not S.[3] Peter, whiche forsoke worldly thinges, but rather sathan, whiche would haue giuen Christe muche riches to haue honored him. But the landes of Princes are too heauie to be caried with his porters, and also too hotte to be troden vpon of anie of his messengers; his net is verie good to catche the great Papist[4] withall, to store the Popes holie pondes at Rome: this net is the inquisition.[5]

The Popes almosededes.

Popes porters.

Vxor.

I will aske but on or two questions; and now our diner is redie. I praie you what meaneth yonder shepherd to clip the sheepe so nere that he bleedeth? it is well painted.

Ciuis.

It semeth a coueteous land Lorde, that doe so oppresse the tenaunt with fines,[6] rents, bribes, &c., whereby he and his familie dooe liue in great miserie like slaues, with continuall penurie and affliction of mynde, and he will neuer suffer the wolle too growe to the full staple, at length to his owne decaie.

Coueltous landelords.

Vxor.

What meaneth yonder foole, that stand upon the tree and cutteth the arme thereof[7] asonder wherevpon he standeth with a sharpe axe, and is fallyng doune hymselfe?[7]

A foole.

---

[1] Ed. 1564, his. [2] Ed. 1564, haue. [3] Omitted in ed. 1564.
[4] Ed. 1564, Oncle.
[5] The words 'this net is the inquisition' are omitted in ed. 1564.
[6] Ed. 1564, fine, rent, bribe, &c. [7] Omitted in ed. 1564.

Ciuis.

Under this[1] predicament is comprehended all traitors against princes, children against Parentes, seruauntes against Maisters, poore against rich, tenauntes against their[2] lordes, &c.; therupon[3] thei doe liue and haue their staie in this worlde, and will seeke their hurtes, whiche in deede is their owne decaie, losse, and destruction in the ende.

Vxor.

Good God! what meaneth that bloudie, naked picture, with a sharpe Rodde in eche hande, woundyng his bodie, and spoyled of all his apparell? *Rebels and knaues.*

Ciuis.

God sende peace in the christen realmes, good Susan,[4] that do signifie by the circumstaunce of some old, wise Painter, that when the bodie and state of anie Realme or realmes of vicinitie, or nerenes together; being as handes to one bodie, or helpers to eche other; If thei bee at strief, the whole bodie wherupon thei are deriued, shall eftesones through the same be ruinated and brought into perill. In this matter I will talke no further as now.[5] *Peace and vnitie God sende us.*

Vxor.

Husbande, in this fine border is curiously painted a house, builded of stone, and with manie strong doores and windowes, barred and railed with strong yron barres; And before one of the doores standyng a man[6] in a plaine poore coate, with white sleues, and a little bodie[7] standyng behinde hym with a faire goune in his armes, Marchaunt like, in a fine blacke cappe; and ouer the dore is written, *Veritas non querit angulos.* I knowe not the meanyng. *Ludgate. Make shifts.*

Ciuis.

In deed, truthe seketh no corners, as these euill disposed, vile Theeues doe, although it was ment to helpe some honest decaied

---

[1] Ed. 1564, that. [2] Omitted in ed. 1564.
[3] Ed. 1564, whereupon; ed. 1573, whervpon. [4] Ed. 1564, good dame.
[5] Ed. 1564 adds 'let vs go to diner a Gods name. Roger, what good felowe is here, to kepe me and your maistres company.'
[6] Ed. 1564 adds 'with a yelow cappe.'
[7] Ed. 1564, and a little boie standeth behinde hym.

citizens, that thei should not bee vtterlie destroied of pitilesse creditours, but after thei might rise up againe; now the bankeroote is in duraunce, hath lost his credence; hee is in prison, where as his credence is spoiled and gone: no man will trust him. But that inne hath a priuiledge to increase manie gestes by this meanes, that thei maie haue libertie with a little aplesquire, to be his keper, or agree with the keeper of the place,[2] which chaungeth his apparell and countinaunce, crepyng into corners, making bargaines in Blackewelhaule,[3] takyng vp euery[4] commoditie, refusyng nothyng: all is fishe that commeth to the nette; he setteth hande and seale to euerything, he sweareth he would not lose his credence for thousandes, hee geueth swete wordes, he knauishly robbeth, undoeth, spoileth the widdowe and the honeste pitifull countreman[5] or true citizen; and when he hath vndoen theim, he runneth to his place againe, as the Fox dooeth to his hole, and liues[6] by the spoile.

Seignior shiftes.[1]
Happy priuilege and subtle practise.
Perillous thieuish bank routes.

Vxor.

What meaneth this straunge picture? Here standeth a manne double, or in twoo, twinnes back to back; the one side is lustie, faire, riche, and yonge, and beautiful; the other side seemeth sicke, foule, poore, and olde; in the yong mannes hande was a grashopper, and in the old mannes an Ant without feete?

Yong & folishe, olde and beggerlie.

Ciuis.

In that table is liuely declared mankinde, both the tyme of his youth, in felicitie, with the careless grashopper, gatheryng nothing; but spoileth house, lande, &c., in bankettes, vice, apparell, and harlottes, &c.; and when age commeth hee would be thryftie, and then can get no more then the lame footeles ante. Then maketh he exclamation, saiyng, oh! what gooddes did my father leaue mee; what good counsaill my frendes gaue me; but I esteemed none of theim both, but in fine lost

A wretche that refused good counsaile in tyme.

[1] Ed. 1564, shifters.   [2] Ed. 1564 omits 'or agree .... piace.'
[3] Ed. 1564, bargaines in euery place.   [4] Omitted in eds. 1573, 1578.
[5] Ed. 1564, marchaunte.   [6] Ed. 1564, liueth.

both riches and frendes, and now I am in great pouertie, sicknes, and age. Lette other men take example by mee, and remember the wisedome of Salomon, saiyng : *Vade ad formicum* [sic] *ô piger et considera vias eius et disce sapientiam,* &c. Goe thou, idle bodie, to the Ante ; consider, and marke well her waies, and learne wisedome ; she hath no guide, prince, nor law geuer, but gathereth in somer to kepe her in winter, &c.

_{A lesson for a lubber.}

Vxor.

There is also painted a lustie yong man, stouping doune to a vessell, in which swimmeth bothe Eles and Snakes; he seemeth to catche one of them: what meaneth that?

Ciuis.

Ha, ha, ha! it is merrily[1] handled; forsothe, it is one that is ouer come either with loue or coueteousnesse. He goeth a woyng, my dyng, dyng; and if he spedeth, my dearlyng, what getteth he, my swetyng? Forsoth, either a serpente that will styng hym all his life with cruell wordes, or els a[2] swete harte with pleasunt speache, that when hee thinketh her moste sure, hee hath but a quicke Ele: you knowe where. Ha, ha, ha! _{Wel fished.[3]}

_{Of a wower how he sped.}

Vxor.

There[4] standeth a manne in comely, faire attire, like vnto purple in Graine, A longe purse by his girdle, and a chaine of golde about his necke. He hath a Lyon in a chaine on the one side, and a Fox in a slippe on the other side; it is a trim picture, well painted.

Ciuis.

Thus goeth it with the worlde, that where as menne by crafte and flatterie of the Foxe can not deceiue the poore widow and fartherlesse, as often tymes thei do, good Susan; then most cruellie, with violence, they use the forse of the Lion, with greuous wronges, extortion, and violence; neither regardyng the goodes, teares, or liues of them whom thei doe oppresse, nor

_{Eccle. v. Eccle. liii. Abacu. i. a.}

---

[1] Eds. 1573, 1578, merely.   [2] Omitted in ed. 1564.
[3] Eds. 1573, 1578, finished.
[4] 'There standeth ... Aske me no more questions, good Susan' (p. 94) omitted in ed. 1564.

Gods curse. This is a pitifull case, marke it well. That when God doeth laie on his crosse, as by the death of the housebande, how is the widowe handled, and the fatherlesse, &c. Doe not the wicked put to their handes with robberie, and thei whiche flattered the father with the Fox, will destroie the sonne with the Lyon.

Vxor.

Who is he that sitteth betweene twoo stooles in that corner?

Ciuis.

This felowe would serue two maisters; his name is Jacke indiffierent, twoo faces in a hoode. He beareth fire in one Apoca. xx. hande, and water in an other; a Papiste and a Protestante, God and Mammon; the Alcaron of Mahomite is as good to hym as the Bible of Christe. The childe when he thinketh hymselfe moste surely sette, then falleth he sonest to the grounde. Bothe his maisters will slippe from hym; he is spewed forthe for that he is neither hotte nor colde.

Vxor.

There is painted a sober, modeste, and a comely picture; in his right hande a Cuppe of fine golde, and in the lefte hande an olde ragged garment: what meaneth this?

Ciuis.

This is an excellent inuention, and thus it is alluded verie well to the saiyng of the wiseman, admonishyng all men with these woordes: Vse well the tyme of prosperitie, and remember the tyme of misfortune; for God, saieth he, maketh the one by the other, So that a man can finde nothyng els under the Sonne.

Vxor.

What beaste is that hauyng many colours, one bodie, and seuen horrible heddes?

Ciuis.

The bodie of sinne with many infernall heddes: wickednesse in euery place under the Sonne.

Vxor.

What ship is that with so many owers and straunge tacle? it is a great vessele?

A DIALOGVE.

Ciuis.

This is the ship of fooles, wherin saileth bothe Spirituall and Temporall of euery callyng. Some there are Kynges, Queenes, Popes, Archbishoppes, Prelates, Lordes, Ladies, Knightes, Note this well. Gentlemen, Phisicions, Lawiers, Marchauntes, Housebandemen, Beggers, theeues, hores, knaues, &c. This ship wanteth a good Pilot, the storme, the rocke, and the wrecke at hand, all will come to naught in this Hulke for want of good gouernement.

Vxor.

What nomber of men in harnesse are these? Some sleapyng, and many of theim semeth to goe wisperyng together, and behind them there appereth other men putting forth their heddes out of corners wearyng no harnesse.

Ciuis.

These are not only the Constables with the watchmen in London, but also almoste through this realme, moste falsely abus- <small>Constables and their watche.</small> yng the tyme, commyng verie late to the watche, sitting doune in some common place of watchyng, wherein some falleth on slepe by the reason of labour or muche drinkyng before, or els nature requireth reste in the night. These fellowes thinke euery hower a thousande vntill thei goe home, home, home, euery man to bed. God night, God night! God saue the Queene! saieth the constables, farewell, neighbours. Eftesones after their departyng creepeth forthe the wilde roge and his fellowes, hauyng two or three other harlottes for their tourne, with picklockes, handesawes, longe Hookes, ladders, &c., to breake into houses, robbe, murther, steale, and doe all mischief in the houses of true men, vtterly vndoyng honest people to maintain their harlottes; greate hoses, lined clokes, long daggers, and feathers, these muste be paid for, &c. This commeth for want of punishment by the daie, and idle watche in the night. God graunt that some of the watche be not the scoutes to the theues. Yes; God graunt that some men haue not conspiratours of Theues in their owne houses, whiche, like Judasses, deciue their maisters. If this watche bee not better looked vnto, good wife, in euery place in this realme, and all the night long searchyng euery suspected corner, no man shall be able to keepe a penie, no scant his owne life in a while. For thei that dare attempt suche 4 matters in the citie of London, what will they doe in houses smally garded, or by the high waie? Yet there is muche execution, but it helpeth not, it is the eccesse of apparell. Hose, hose! great hose! too little wages, too many seruing men, too many tipplyng houses, too 8 many drabbes, too many knaues, too little labour, too muche idlenes.

Vxor.

Jesus, Jesus! good husband, but one question, and then to diner. What are all these, two and two in a table? Oh, it is trim.

12 *Ciuis.*

These are old frendes; it is well handled, and workemanly. Willyam Boswell in Paternoster rowe painted them. Willyam Boswell, a Painter. Here is Christ and Sathan, sainct Peter and Symon 16 Magus, Paule and Alexander the Copersmith, Trace and Becket, Martin Luther and the Pope, Ecolampadius and Fisher, sir Thomas Moore and Jhon Frith, bishop Cranmer and bishop Gardiner, Boner wepyng, Bartlet grene breche, Galen and Gregory Wisedom, Auicen 20 and George Salthous, Salomon and Will Sommer, The George Salthous. Cocke and the Lyon, the Wolfe and the Lambe, and thus I doe ende. Aske me no more questions, good Susan.

Roger.

24 Sir, there is one lately come into this Inne[1] in a greene Kendall coate, with yellowe hose, a bearde of the same colour, onely upon the upper lippe, a balde chin,[2] a russet hatte, with a greate plume of straunge feathers, and a braue scarffe about his necke, in cutte 28 buskens. He is plaiyng at the treatrip[3] with our hoste Mendax is described. sonne; he plaieth tricke vpon the Gitterne, and daunce Trenchemore and Hey de Gie, and telleth newes from Terra Florida. He looketh a squinte, he daunceth vp and doune;[4] I did see him

---

[1] Ed. 1564, hall.   [2] Ed. 1564 omits 'a balde chin.'
[3] Eds. 1564, 1573, trea trippe.
[4] 'he daunceth vp and doune' omitted in ed. 1564.

giue the good man a pece of a Unicornes horne good against poison; he semeth a pretie scholer. But I heard hym praie the chamberlain in his eare to lende him vi^d upon a pressing yron, which chamberlain refused the gage. 4

Ciuis.

Roger, call hym to[1] dinner, it is some pleasaunte fellowe, and laketh money; be like through trauaile the poore man is driuen to his shiftes, and would make other men merie   Well taken.   8
when he weepeth in his owne[2] harte.

Vxor.

Good housebande, call in some graue companie. What should suche Jackes and tospottes dooe here? He semeth to   A good wife.   12
be some theef or ruffin. Fie on hym, verlet, fie, fie!

Roger.

By our Ladie, I will fetche hym into diner; he is a good companion for me. Wee shall heare newes.   News.   16

Ciuis.

Goe thy waies quickly.

Roger.

Sir, my maister and my maistres praie your Maistershippe to 20
take the paines to come to their chamber, whereas you   A gentle gretyng.
shal be hartely welcome to their dinner.

Mendax.

Sir, I will waite upon them, but first I will vpon this whetstone 24
sharpe my knife.

Roger.

Sir, here is this gentleman come to keep you companie.

Ciuis.   28

He is moste hartely welcome, set hym a chaire; giue him a trencher and a napkin. I praie you take parte of suche as God hath sente; if it were at London I might make you better chere, but here I cannot.   32

[1] Ed. 1564, into.   [2] Omitted in ed. 1564.

A DIALOGVE.

Mendax.

Here is good cheare; I was there within these ten weekes that I would haue giuen twentie shillynges for suche a loafe as this, whereas no suche cheare was to be had. *Mendax doe beginne.*

Ciuis.

Where was it,[1] I praie you, gentle maister? I cannot tell what to call you, nor of what countrie you are.

Mendax.

Sir, I was borne nere vnto Tunbridge, where fine kniues are made; my name is *Mendax*, a yonger brother linially descended of an auncient house before the conquest. We giue three Whetstones in Gules with no difference, and vpon our creste a lefte hand, with a horne uppon the thombe, and a knife in the hande. The supporters are a Foxe on th' one side, and a Frier on the other side. And of late I traueiled into Terra Florida, whereas I felt both wealth and woe; the blacke oxe neuer trode vpon my foote before, a dogge hath but a daie. We are borne al to trauaile, and as for me I haue but little to lose, yet I am a gentleman, and cannot find in my harte to plaie the slaue, or go too cart; I neuer could abide it, by the masse. *Mendax, his armes.* *A Ruffian.*

Ciuis.

You speake like a wiseman. I perceiue by your behauioure that you haue been well brought vp. I praie you, where is that land? *Ironia.*

Mendax.

Many M[2] miles beyonde Torrida Zona, on the Equinoctiall line, in the Longitude nere vnto the Pole Antartike; it is an C.M.[3] miles long, and is in the part named America; and by the waie are the Islandes called Fortunato or Canaria, whose west partes be situated in the thirde Climate. *Terra Florida described by maister Mendax.*

Ciuis.

It was a daungerous trauaile into that countrie; where landed you? At what place?

---

[1] Eds. 1564, 1573, that. [2] Ed. 1564, C. [3] Ed. 1565, xvij. M.

Mendax.

Wee sailed to the Islandes of Portum Sanctum, and then to Medera, in whiche were sondrie countrees and islandes, as Eractelentie, Magnefortis, Grancamarie, Tenereffe, Palme Ferro, &c. And our captaine went with his Soldiours to lande. And at our first commyng nere vnto the Riuer in one of these Islandes, as we refreshed our selues emong the Date trees, in the lande of Palmes, by the sweete welles, we did, to the greate feare of vs all, se a great battaile betwene the Dragon and the Vnicorne;[1] and, as God would, the vnicorne thrust the dragon to the hart; and, againe, the dragon with his taile stong the vnicorne to death. Here is a peece of his horne; the blood of dragons is riche; the[2] battaile was worth 200 markes to our capitain. *A battaile very proffitable.* Then we traueiled further into Teneriffa, into an exceedyng high mountaine, aboue the middle region, wheras we had greate plentie of roche[3] Alom, And might well heare an heauenly Hermonie emong the Starres. The moone was nere hand vs with marueilous heate; and *He was near the Starres.* when we came doune at the hill foote growe many grosse herbes, as Louage, Laserpitium, Acanthus and Solanum; and whether it was by the eatyng of Solanum or no, there was a greate[4] mightie man naked and hearie, in a deepe slepe, whom wee gently suffered too lye still. He had a greate beard in which a birde did breede, and brought her younge ones meate; this[5] man slepte halfe a yere, and waked not. Our capitain declared vnto vs *no lie, no lie.* that the spials had vewed the lande, and how that our enemies were at hande. The next daie moste fearfull people painted with sondry colours approached in strange beastes skinnes, with Flint so were their shaftes and dartes made,[6] with whom wee fought and slewe, and tooke some, and yet the people so assaulted vs, that with much difficultie wee recouered our Barkes; and then wee sailed forthe, and chaunced to let fal our sounding lead newe tallowed, whervpon did sticke gold. With all spede we sent doune our diuers, and so within three daies we gathered thirtie hogsheddes of fine gold, besides twoo

---

[1] Eds. 1573, 1578, Vnicore. [2] Eds. 1564, 1573, that.
[3] 'roche' omitted in ed. 1564. [4] Ed. 1564, verie mightie.
[5] 'this man ... waked not' omitted in ed. 1564.
[6] Ed. 1564 omits 'made.'

buttes of orient perles; al the shore was full of currall. From thence wee sailed to the greate Isle called Madagasta,[1] in Scorea, where were Kynges, Mahumitaines by religion, blacke as deuilles. Some had no heddes, but eyen in their breastes. Some, when it rained, couered all the whole bodie with one foote. That[2] land did abound in Elephantes teeth; the men did eate Camiles and Lions fleshe. Muske and Zeuet in euery place did abounde, and the mother of perle, wherof[3] the people made their platters to put in their meate; thei dwell emong spice; the ground is moiste with oile of precious trees. Plenty of wine out of grapes as big as this lofe; muche Peper; thei cannot tell what to doe with Suger; but that their marchauntes of Maabar, twentie daies iourney of, doe come and take of their gooddes franckly for nothyng; but some of them do bryng yron to make edge tooles, for which thei haue for one pounde twentie[4] pounde of fine gold; their pottes, pannes, and all vessell are[5] cleane gold garnished with Diamondes. I did see swine feede in them.

Mendax bringeth good tidynges of treasure and richesse, and where it is.

Ciuis.

Did you se no strange foules there and fishes?

Mendax.

In the isle called Ruc, in the great Cans lande, I did see Marmaides and Satyres with other fishes by night, came fower miles from the sea, and climed into trees, and did eate dates and nutmegges, with whom the Apes and Babians had muche fightyng, yelling, and criyng. The people of the land do liue by eating the fleshe of women. In this land did I se an Ape plaie at Ticketack, and after at Irishe on the tables with one of that lande; And also a Parate giue one of their gentlewomen a checkmate at Chesse. There[7] Gese daunce Trenchmore.

The beste meate and the worste.[6]

Ciuis.

God keepe us[8] from those cruell people.

---

[1] 'Madagastat' in Ed. 1573.   [2] Ed. 1564, The.
[3] 'wherof' omitted in ed. 1564.   [4] Ed. 1564, twelve.   [5] Ed. 1564, is.
[6] Ed. 1564, worste meate.   [7] 'There ... Trenchmore' omitted in ed. 1564.
[8] Ed. 1564, me.

Mendax.

But, sir, as for Birdes, thei are not onely infinit in numbers, but also in kindes; Some voyces moste sweete, and some moste fearfull; Nightingales as bigge as Gese, Oules greater then some horse; and there are birdes that doe lye in a rocke where Dragons are, whose Feathers on[1] their wynges are thirtie foote long, the quill as bigge as a canon roiall; also I heard Parates dispute in Philosophie, Freshe in Greke, and[2] sing discant. Also there are a people called Astomis,[3] which liue very long, and neither eat nor drinke, but onely liue by ayre and the smell of fruites. In Selenetide there are women, contrary to the nature of other women, doe laie egges, and hatche them from whom doe children come 1. 12 tymes greater then those which are borne of women. There did I see Scipodes hauyng but one foote, whiche is so broad that thei couer all their bodies for the raine and the Sonne.

Item, I did see men hauyng feete like horse, called Ipopodes.

Item, I did see the Satyres halfe men and halfe Goates plaiyng vpon Cornets.

Item, I did se Apothami, halfe horse and halfe man.

Item, I plaied at tables with the people called Fanesis,[4] whose eares were as long as clokes, coueryng all their bodies; nere them is the great citie called O, iiij.c. miles within the wall; the wall was Brasse, twoo M gates, sixe C bridges as bigge as London bridge; the Citie paued with golde. Naked menne dwell there with twoo heades and six handes euery man. There did I se apes plaie at Tennis.

Ciuis.

I praie you is there any plentie of precious stones?

Mendax.

Verie many, but harde to come by; but in the island Zanzibar is muche plentie of Ambergrise, that thei make claie for their houses withall; there, if wee had holden together like frendes, we might haue gotten a worlde.[5] When[6] I

Birdes of straunge kindes.

Ambergrise as plentifull as claie.

---

[1] Ed. 1573, in.
[2] 'and sing discant . . . apes plaie at Tennis' omitted in ed. 1564.
[3] Ed. 1573, Astomij.   [4] Ed. 1573, Fanesij.   [5] Ed. 1564, a great kingdome.
[6] Ed. 1564, O my hart! it maketh it blede when, &c.

doe remember it, alas,[1] alas, euery man is but for hymself; you maie consider what diuision is; Emeroddes, Rubbies, Turkies, Diamondes, & Saphiers were solde when we came thether first for the waighte of yron; a M riche Turkesses were solde for iijs iiijd;[2] to bee shorte, one with another, after iijs iiijd a pecke. Our men gather[3] vp Carbuncles and Diamondes with rakes under the spice trees. *Precious stones moste plentifull.* *Diamondes gathered with rakes.*

Ciuis.

How chaunce you brought none home in to this realme.

Mendax.

Oh, sir, wee filled twoo shippes with fine gold, three shippes with Ambergrise, Muske, and Vnicornes hornes, and twoo tall Barkes, with precious stones, and sailed by the Adamante stones, which will drawe yron vnto theim, and so caste awaie the greatest riches in Heathenes or Christendome. After that cruell chaunce we came vppon the maine lande of Cuba, in the greate and mightie lande of America, where as the people called Canabals do dwel in caues, rockes, and woodes; there as women will eate their owne children, and one man an other, and thei are Gyantes moste high and fearfull, all goe naked; the[i] neither knowe good humanitie, humaine policie, religion, lawe, nor chastitie. One is equal with another, the strongest of bodie are chifest, for there al is ruled by force and not through reason, after the maner of Swine. Children loue their fathers no more than Pigges doe the Bores, for thei saie luste causeth generation. And when their parentes are very old thei bryng them to an exceading high mountain, where as is a greate tower builded vpon a Rocke, vnder whiche tower is the golden Myne, in which Myne there bee twoo greate monstrous dragons kepyng the same, which wil neuer suffer the children to come to receiue the benefites of that place vntil such tyme as thei haue slaine their parentes, and cast their flesh into the caue, and washe[d] the dragons Image which are within that tower, made of precious wood, with the *A great loss, it hath undon all England.* *Cruel women.* *A good commonweath.* *The price of golde.*

---

[1] Ed. 1564 omits 'alas, alas.'   [2] Ed. 1564, for iiij. d.
[3] Ed. 1564, gathered.

bloud of their saied parentes. From whence[1] we traueiled into an island, where as it neuer raineth but once a yere, and that is in the moneth of July, whereas Nilus runneth by giuyng benefit vnto the plaine countrie, whereas spice of all kindes doeth growe. In that Island doeth growe Apples[2] most plentifully, whiche thei dooe call Lupilum. A little before our commyng was a greate winde, whiche had shaken doune muche fruite and precious spice, and many hundred carte loades of good Hoppes. After whiche fell doune plentie of raine, raisyng a myghtie floud, incontinent succeded a burnyng heate, for it is vnder the Equinoctial line or Torrida Zona. In fine, throwe this coniunction[3] of the Sonne mouing this boilyng of the water, through the help of muche spice, I neuer dranke suche Hipocras wine nor Beere; the Flemynges haue founde out the commoditie and caren to transport no more Hoppes hether vnto us. And if good lucke had been our[4] lord, we had made our selues and all the christian kingdomes for euer.

A miracle of double Bere.

Where it remaineth [raineth] double Bere.

A feaste for Flemynges.

Ciuis.

Alas, alas, what was that? I pray you tell me. I am sory that you and your frendes haue traueiled thus long, and haue been in daunger for nothing. But I perceiue you haue been a greate traueiler, and haue seen many countries, woodes, and riuers.

Mendax.

Non finis erit si prosequar omnia verbis,
Flumina et specos, campos, siluasque lacusque,
Colles, apricosque siunosque undeque portus,
Omnia sunt vidi. Now let them go,
I haue seen those thynges and manie moe.

Loquax

Syr, in the landes beyond *Cuba* or as the Cosmographars cal *Lamiam* or *Ianicam*, whereas the people doe curse the Sunne at noone because it burneth them, there[5] is a fletyng Island swymming about the sea, by what meanes I knowe not, whether occasioned by Corcke, Wooll, &c.; it woulde by the winde shifte from place to place. Sume saied

A new land that swimmeth, commyng from Paradise.

---

[1] Eds. 1564, 1573, thence. [2] Ed. 1564, hoppes.
[3] Ed. 1564, concoction. [4] Ed. 1564, our good lord.
[5] Ed. 1564, there are many Islands emong them, there is, &c.

it was a shred of the bankes of Paradise, broken through the force of Ganges, and so in continuance brought downe. It was not brode. In that Isle were but fewe people. And the menne of that place doe
4 by proper art, with a sharp flint stone, worme the women, <small>Women with wormes in their tongues.</small> and pretely cut their tongues, and take forth a smale Serpente aliue, and heale their Tongues agayne with herbe grace. The[1] Italians make poysons of this Serpent. This Island hath many riche
8 stones, gold and spice in it, with precious trees, as Agallicum and Guiacum. In that Isle there had been some Frenche men, <small>Guiacum.</small> whose skinnes were clene cast of in the maner of Snakes; marie, they were full of hooles. This Guiacum did much pleasure to them belike.
12 But as wee were deuising howe to steale this lande awaie, and bryng it forthe to the maine Sea with our Pilottes twoo thinges <small>A great loss.</small> letted our purpose. The one was the Hauen mouthe was to straighte, the second the people were to vigilant and letted our purpose. But I
16 truste I and my companions will make oue lustie voyage, and geue an onset, for all wee will either winne the saddle[2] or loose the horse. We are none but good fellowes; of my parte, I will doe what lieth in me to make menie prentises free, and cause other good yong <small>Honest fellowe</small>
20 Gentlemen in sellyng their land to get thousandes. If men knewe as muche as I dooe in this matter, they had rather venter the best ioynt then be from thence, it is almoste heauen; and if we do wante by the waye, let euery man kepe close, and there we maie
24 chaunce to find some little fleting Islandes,[3] wherein <small>Pirates, heires of Wapping for their snapping.</small> good Suger, Spice, Silke, Linnen, &c.,[4] readie made, and that will make readie money, and money maketh a man. Oh, that young menne woulde beleue me, and followe me, I woulde make
28 theym Lordes or K.[5]

[1] 'The ... serpent' omitted in ed. 1564.   [2] So ed. 1564; ed. 1573, sandle.
   [3] Ed. 1564, adds 'by the waie.'   [4] Ed. 1564, adds 'do growe.'
    [5] Ed. 1564, omits 'or K,' and proceeds thus:—

Vxor.
Good housebande, hearken in your eare. I would speake with you, swete harte.
Ciuis.
Speake on youre mynde, good Susan. What is the matter, woman?
Vxor.
Sir, this is a blinde iyed shameles ruffen, a roge, I warrante hym, and

Ciuis.
Were you euer in the lande of *Ethiopia* ?

Mendax.
I knowe all that lande; it is an exeedyng greate lande. It is from the *Equinoctial* towarde the Pole Antartike, and is deriued both of Asia and Affrike; neere the famous Reuer, runnyng through the Islande & the long mountaines called *Luna*. Prester Ihon do dwell in the east parte. The chiefest citie is called *Meroa*, some- tyme *Saba*. The Queene of that Citie came to Salomon. I did see him toumbed in *Meroa*, nere hande as brode and as long as Westminster Haule, made of pure Christall and Golde, garnished with costly Saphires and Diamondes, xx pound waight euerie stone. Through the whiche Christall, whosoeuer had eaten of the herbe called *Apium risum*, growynge in the land *Lekthyophages*, where as the people doe bewitche eche other; then fower houres in the night, through the Christall, one may se King Salomon, Quene Saba, & .iiij.c. ladies daunsing with noble graces in riche attyre, with garlandes of roses on their heddes; and round about the inwarde border of the tombe manie[1] Seraphins with Lutes, Citrons and Harpes plaiyng a thefe. This knaue is hable to make children run from their parentes, seruauntes robbe their maisters, yong heires to sell their landes, men to run from their wiues, and women also. You maie knowe by his Armes of what stocke he cometh; I warrant him from drouning and diying of the Pestilence. Oh, villaine, he wilbe hanged. I dare saie he knoweth al kindes of theues, vagabondes, rouers & hasarders. I like not his words nor his braggyng countenance. Let vs hence.

She describeth a ruffian.

Ciuis.
Well, moche good doe you; you haue taken moche paine, but smalle profite; you haue trauailed farre and maie speake by aucthoritee. Come, take awaie: paie the reconyng. Roger, horse, horse, and awaie!

Roger.
All thynges are readie, sir.

Well rid of euill store.

Ciuis.
Fare ye well, gentle frende.

Mendax.
I thanke you of your gentle companie, good gentleman.

Vxor.
Whose faire fielde is yonder, &c. [Continuing as on p. 112.]

[1] Ed. 1573, maie,

with greate joye. In the ende, Salomon, as his daiely maner was, kissed only the Quene, and saluted the Ladies, so the Ladies with the Cherubens vanished awaie, and Salomon laie downe by the Queene vpon a riche bedde, and they twoo did sleepe there. Betwene whom there was a red hande holdyng a long naked Sworde, to guide the Queene, for feare of the thyng that you wot of. This did I see by my troth. Now a little more of the walles. They vse their magike by stones, wordes, and herbes; with herbes of hot kyndes I haue seen them transforme men into Lyons and Wolues, and manie Womenne into Sowes, she Goates and Apes. With moyste herbes, men into fishes, and women into Apletrees. And in Somer the trees full of Aples, and sodainly by a secret hid *Antypothia*, these Apples are all transformed into children aliue, and grow a pace, as Barnacles dooe in Scotlande, whiche barnacles do growe vpon trees by the Sea side. So doe their children in some places there, but not euerie where, of this cometh it to passe that the *Anthropophager* are desirous to eate of eche other through these Enchauntmentes and coniuringes; of all flesh they doe loue the Coniurers flesh, and all their kynd, as example. The holie house of the Enquisiters of Spain sente into that lande of late one hundredth Friars, commaundyng them onely, accordyng to the Romishe rules, to set up Aulters at their arriual; and so say masse in their holie golden clothes, and so they did. But when the Canabales spied their bald pates, and also their coniuringes, neither fearyng Deuell nor Pope that sent theim, without anye scruple of conscience they did eate them all; and if I, by the eating of an herbe called *Dorademus*, which a witch taught me, had not been turned into a Dogge, I had been eaten of them also, and in thende, by good hap, I fed vpon the knaue Friers bones six dayes. My boy was so stronglie bewitched that he is a dogge still. This same is he; he was a gentleman of a good house; he vnderstandeth vs well, and sometyme was a proper man, and shoulde haue maried with one in London called Ione Trim : whiche nowe are, God wot, of sondrie kyndes, but differ not in conditions, chast, religious, and kynd harted. When I departed from the Canabales Then I ranne from Isle to Isle, and came through a lande of fire called Hell : it was full of burnynge Salamanders, no more hurte

A DIALOGVE. 105

with fire then fishes are with water. Indeede, a Witche led me
through there. I did see and heare many of mine olde acquaintaunce, but thei did not see me; shee tolde me in her language it was
purgatory, sayng thus, *Irepop Si Ireuank sina a yel*. Then came
I into the Lande of *Parthalia*, whiche is a lande of Giantes, tall men,
sum one hundreth foote long, and verie olde; the guide, by interpretation, tolde mee that one was aliue there whiche was a labourer of
Rome when it was firste builded. I did see hym shake xxi bushelles
of Oysters from the tree wheras Oysters do growe, which tree was a
slight shoote of hight; this was aliue Anno 1562. Then came I
iust upon our Antipodie, foote against foote, in a land like ours, and
al had been in one climate, of Riuers, Hilles, and Valies like ours.
There is Gaddes hill, Stangate hole, Newe Market heath, like ours in
all pointes; Also countries like Wales, Tinsdale and Riddesdale;
sauing there were some true men but here is scant one in them, I
trowe, in Tinsdale.

Roger.

I praie you honeste man surreuerence you; cleane felow masse
mendhouse, is there any greate Citie in that land?

Mendax.

Goodman *Loquax*, my name is not masse mendhouse; I am no
Carpenter. My name is *Mendax*, whiche in the *Ethiope* tongue
signifieth the name of a greate Citie, the mother of holie religion &
truth, and is called *Emor*, in maners like *Modos* & *Romog*.

Ciuis.

Is there any greate Citie?

Mendax.

I, forsoth, there is one old famous Citie of a great antiquitie, the
best reformed Citie of this woorlde; the like hath not been hard of,
neither red of, nor seen. Barbarous Grekes cal it in their language
Metonoyæ, whiche by interpretation in their tongue is called *Ecnat-
neper* or *Nodnol*. The land is called *Taerg Natrib*, a most auncient
land, and Christians all sworne enemies to the Pope.

Ciuis.

I praie you howe is the Citie reformed?

Mendax.

I will beginne first of their Saboth daie, whiche is the seuenth daie, that is sondaie; and as thei doe in this hedde Citie, so all the other Cities doe. Townes and Villages all dooe the same, for I doe knowe theym all, for in that land are 1560 parish Churches. Sometyme they had manie horrible dennes of Idolatrie called *Seiabba*, verie riche, whose landes the wise Princes gaue, and changed euen to some of the temporall priestes, and which haue suche swetenes in the riches and gaine thereof. Although that many of theim doe loue Papistrie, thei had rather the Citie of Rome with the Popes holynes were vtterlie burned, yea, and Christes also together, then they woulde loose their Abbaie Landes. Oh, it passeth *Terra Florida*, and yet for all this I thinke they are Protestantes; not one Papiste in all that lande, I warrante you; no, nor one wicked liuer.

Ciuis.

Tushe man to the matter concerning the kepyng of the Saboth daie tell that to the ende; and then a reckning with our hostes, and let vs departe, it is three of clocke smitten; I must awaie; I haue farre to ride this euenyng.

Mendax.

This Citie is greate, well walled, and strongly fortified; warlike, with greate gates, verie beautifull, as euen Hierusalem was. These gates are locked faste vppon the Sabboth, sauyng the small portales, to this ende that the Citizens dooe not goe, neither ride forth of the Citie duryng that daie, except it be after the euenyng praier; then to walke honestlie into the sweete fieldes, and at euery gate in the time of seruice there are warders.

Ciuis.

What, then, will they not suffer the traueilers and countrie dwellers to Iorneye to their townes and dwellyng places?

Mendax.

No, surely, not one; but that[1] so euer hee be he muste kepe hollie the Sabboth daie, and come to the churche, both man, woman, yong and olde.

Ciuis.

It is not possible; who do loke to the yonge children, sicke folkes, and make prouision for diner and supper?

Mendax.

This is the matter; in euerie Churche they haue two worthie ministers, for there are no pluralities. These men are knowen to be wise, sober, honeste, and learned; the better learned is the Preacher, the other dooe minister the Sacramentes; and both of these haue good stipendes, and greate reuerence done to theim. They doe shewe suche light to the blinde, thei visite the sick, they moue people to pitie the poore, and forgeue their enemies; and at the sounde of the bell the seruauntes and such as muste attende at home when their maisters dooe come from the Church, at the seconde Sermond all here the first Sermon, wheras thei doe beginne to sing with holie Psalmes before the Sermond and also after. And after the Communion is done they soborlie departe, geuyng attendance, that the familie at home of the yong children or sicke be deligentlye looked vnto, prouidyng the diner for their masters, &c., whiche are present at the second Sermonde with their wiues, &c. Oh, blessed sight! the heauenliest meeting that euer was seen or hearde with mortall eyen or eares; would God that I were there againe! There is not one Usurer: not one.

Ciuis.

Why, what sight it is, I praie you, or what hearyng that is so heauenly?

Mendax.

There is no mingled doctrine, no tromperie of Papistrie, but the naked, true, and perfite worde of God. No flattering in the preacher, neither railing, but teaching truly euery manne his duetie to God, their prince and one to another; the greate curses of the lawe, and

---

[1] Ed. 1573, what.

sweete promises of the Gospel. There is excommunication of the vngodly, Discipline to the penitentes, and godly reconciliation again into the Churche, openly confessyng their faultes, makyng restitution of wronges, breakyng the othes of wicked bargaines, hauyng the greate feare of Iudgement of God before their eyen, whiche maketh theim to tremble; doyng no wronge one vnto an other, neither by extortion, vsurie, euill ware sold by vntruth for good, &c. With collections of money for the poore in deede; the idle are sette to woorke or sore punished for slothe. Is not this well doen, maister *Ciuis* ?

Ciuis.

If this be true it is a blessed Citie. How doe they spende the afternoone, I pray you?

Mendax.

Euen as thei did in the fore Noone, the communion excepted, in which place the yong people are examined in the principall partes of the Christen faith. And one thyng did I note in that Cittie, and also in the other,[1] there were no people walking abroad in the seruice tyme; no, not a Dogge or a catte in the streate, neither any Tauerne doore open that daie, nor wine bibbyng in them, but onely almose, fasting, and praier.

Ciuis.

How do they punishe the Sabboth daie breakers, and other offences?

Mendax.

Accordyng to the offence; there is no respecte of persones; there the magistrate is greuously punished as the poore people for geuing euill example.

The drunkarde is punished with fasting in prison certain daies.

The adulterer by death; so is the fellon or murderer accordyng to Moses lawes.

The vnreconciled stubborne againste the parentes are put to death if they be companions by their parentes.

The berwardes are greuously whipped for that outrage with Dogges, Beares, and Apes plaie on the Sabboth daie lyke our bedles.

[1] Ed. 1573, others.

The Juglers eyes are put out.
The common swearer doe lose his tonge.
The Ruffin is chained & whipped like our Bedles.
The double handed Lawier, or double dealer in poore mennes causes is kept in prison, and forfite his goodes to the prince, and the wrongfull oppressed.
The extorcioner is made a begger.
The promoter for his own proper gaine is coumpted a K.
The informer for a Common wealthe is coumpted honest, and well regarded.
The defrauder of the wages of the laborer and seruauntes so proued is in case of Fellonie.
The wilfull periurie [sic] is stoned to death, with tongue cut out.
The knowne peruerse Papiste is burned, for in hym is coumpted a nomber of treasons, as he would the chaung of Religion, The Pope to gouerne the Prince, the destruction of the faithful; Ergo, a traitour, thefe, knaue, &c.

Ciuis.

So Goddes lawes and the Princes are obserued in that happie lande. I praie you what is the cause?

Mendax.

The are written ouer all the Citie gates, and in their Churches in letters limned with golde. The woordes of Christe, sainct Peter, or saincte Paule, *omnes honorate fraternitatem diligite,* 1 Peter 2. *deum timete, regem honorate.* And they haue these wordes written in their hartes and doynges, so their brotherly loue, their feare of God, and the honor of the Prince or Kyng is the cause. The effecte that dooe followe is justice, charite, quietnesse. And so God doe cast his blessing vpon them, ij haruestes in one yeere. The holye Curates make suche peace in their cures that the people goe to no lawe, I warraunt you.

Roger.

Why, are there no theeues? Are not the Lawiers as riche as they are here in our countrie? for here the Lawiers doe swarme as thicke as euer did Friers or Monkes in hell, and be as full of coueteousnesse as euer the Friers were full of superstition.

Mendax.

There was not a robberie, murder, periurie, or any horrible crime committed this xxi. yeres: in this case why should the sworde be drawen? Euery manne doeth knowe his owne, and doe liue in peace, using much fasting and prayer. There are iudges and worthie Lawiers in euerie Cittie whiche haue great stipendes of the prince, & take no fees of the people; not a pynne. They dooe giue counsaile in the countrie freely. They are wise, godlie, & peacemakers; they haue no pettie Foggers, nor a swarme of sedicious disquieters of the common wealth like thieues; no, not like theues, but theeues themselues.

Ciuis.

One question more. Are they at peace with their neighbours of other nations?

Mendax.

Nature hath placed their lande within the Sea, like this lande. That is one garde. Also they haue in store a greate stronge Nauie of shippes well appointed, and all their coastes with Castles, Blockhouses, Beacons, watchemen. Thei haue many famous men of warre, valiaunte, good of iudgemente, and also well trained Soldiours, faithful, hardie, and obedient; euerie one of these can well handle his peece or shoot in a Bowe. Their Capitaines, in the tyme of peace, haue greate wages to maintaine them; it behoueth theim so to maintaine their men of Warre for feare the Golden fleese be stolen. For it is a good Land for Woll and Corne, muche desired of the Enemies; and in the old tyme often runne ouer with other nations. The men there are[1] xx foote hyght.

Mendax would sooner sale the truth.

Ciuis.

How are the people appareled?

Mendax.

Verie plain, sauing the nobles, which are riche, in faire attire like angelles. There the women are verie huswifly, the men homely, greate labor, little silke is worne, no ieuels, no light colours, no great hose, no long daggers, no cockscombe feathers, no double

---

[1] Omitted in ed. 1573.

ruffes, not many seruyng men, no dising nor unlawfull games;
neither coggyng, knauerie, foystyng, or cosenyng. Plaine, plaine;
plain both in word and dede. Muche hospitalitie, speciallie among
the Cleargie; no pride among them, but mercie, mercie, and pittie,
pittie. Also in their courte is no vanitie nor flatterers, but verie
curtesie, and in all pointes ruled by God's word in vnitie.

And thus fare you well, for this is true or els I doe lye.

Roger.

I will sweare vppon a Booke thy laste woordes are true, and all
the reste are lies. You might haue told the tale at Whetston,[1] and
won the beste game; thou went neuer in suche landes, neither hast
thou seen anie such comonwelth. Farewel, goodman knaue.

Ciuis.

Awaie, Roger, fetche forthe my horse. Gentleman, fare you
well, I dooe giue credite to your tale. You muste bere with my
man, he is a verlet, and you a gentleman of great trauel, iudgement,
and experience.

Mendax.

Sir, in your presence I will not deale with hym, for your courteous entertainemente. But as I am true gentleman, as I am in deede,
I will whip the slaue if I doe meete hym alone, for giuyng me the
lye; he doeth me great dishonour; I will not beare it at his handes.
I haue slain aboue .30. for callyng me liyng knaue. God haue
mercie vpon their soules; I am very cholericke.

Ciuis.

Giue me your hande; you shall knowe this shalbe corrected of
my parte, God willyng, who keepe you. Fare you wel. Yet once
again, good Maister *Mendax*, fare ye well.

Mendax.

Fare you well, gentle Maister *Ciuis;* and you, good maistres.

Vxor.

God be out of your waie for stomblyng.

---

[1] Ed. 1573, Wheston.

Roger.

I praie God the Gallowes gnawe thy knaues bones.

Mendax.

4   Well, knaue, well; by the Masse I will not forget you, you vile Roge; I will trim you for this geare if I catche you.

Vxor.

Whose[1] faire fielde is yonder, I woulde faine knowe it, and let
8 trifles passe, I will not beleue theim; let foolishe thynges goe, and talke of matters profitable. *Fair fieldes.*

Roger.

Maistres, doe you not knowe it? It is my Maisters; I am the[2]
12 Bailie there. He had a good bargaine, I assure you; it was a[3] morgage to hym this twoo yeres; I woulde he might finde the like purchesse. All yonder toune is his; he hath raised the rent one hundreth markes a yere more then it was. There were good liyng in the
16 plague time, for there are large pastures, and the houses are doune, sauyng the Manner place, for the carles haue forfected their Leases, and are gone a beggyng like villaines, and many of them are dedde for honger. *Honest landlordes, God amend them!*

20 ### Vxor.

Whose oxen are these, Roger?

Roger.

My maisters also, for he that hath money shall haue lande and
24 worshippe. My maister is a close wiseman, and lieth in the winde of theim that will buye money for lande. *A nette for fooles.*
He can handle a yong gentlemanne trimly, and ride him *A horse maister.*
with a golden snaffle; he knoweth vpon whiche side his breade is
28 buttered well enough, I warrante you. My maister hath risen[4] so earely this mornyng that he noddeth as he rideth.

Vxor.

Sir, me thinkes I doe well perceiue[5] you totter as you ride.
32 What! are you asleepe? Do you not heare your mannes prating?

---

[1] At this point ed. 1564 begins again.   [2] Ed. 1564, his.   [3] Ed. 1564, in.
[4] Ed. 1564, rised.   [5] Ed. 1564 omits 'I do well perceiue.'

He is pleasantely disposed; he would make me beleue that you were a greate landed man, and had muche cattell in store. Why, sir, how doe you that you speake not to me?

Ciuis.

Wife, wife! God sende vs good lucke: do you not see yonder cloude in the Weste towardes the north commyng hether? <small>Feare and dread.</small>

Vxor.

Moste fearfull; God sende vs good lucke. Sir, it is a sodaine chaunge; I will hide my face, it feareth me so muche.

Roger.

I am fourtie yeres olde, but I did neuer se the like but once, and that was betwene Godmichester and Gogmanshille, a little from Cambridge, as I traueiled to Wolpit faire to buye Coltes. And there appeared a straunge forme, as me thought, a greate <small>Roger did see visions.</small> nomber of steples were broken, and manie naked Friers, Bishops, and the Pope hymself, did wryng their handes in ragged clothes; thei looked all very leane: and then it thondered and lightened, <small>A Pittifull case.</small> in whiche storme many Gese were killed, and also shepe and lambes. The yere after was the tumblyng doune of Abbaies, and the reformation of[1] the Churche matters; but this passeth.[2] For the precious passion of Christ let us run awaie with speede. I doe see a fearfull thyng in the cloudes appering, a blacke leane naked bodie, very long, ridyng vpon a pale, miserable foule iade; he hath also <small>Death appeareth with iij dartes.</small> three dartes in his left hande; the one is cole blacke, the other bloud redde, and the third is a darcke pale; he hath no fleshe vppon hym, me thinketh that I doe see a greate fire, and many fearfull monsters in the same followe hym, with a fearfull voice, sayng, All the wicked shall come to vs. Wee are swallowed vp[3] in the seconde death.

Ciuis.

Lette vs take this house: ride apace! the storme doeth begin moste fearfull. God help vs! what shall we doe, or <small>A greate thunder.</small> whether shall wee flie? Jesus, Jesus! what a thonder is this!

---

[1] Ed. 1564, for.   [2] So ed. 1564; eds. 1573, 1578, but let this passe.   [3] Omitted in ed. 1564.

As heauen and yearth should goe together. Lorde, how the lightnyng falleth from heauen! All this region is vpon a flamyng fire; the birdes fall from the trees: loke how the cattell tremble, and trees are
4 pulled vp by the rootes, and the houses are burnte with celestill fire!

Vxor.

Lette vs departe from these trees, for I haue heard saie to sit under a white thorne is most safe and surest in a tempest. <small>Witche crafte.</small>
8 I haue here many goodly ieuelss against lightning, as the Carbuncle, Hemoralde, Hiasinthus, with Amber and Gold. God and S. Barbara defende vs. I haue a S. Ions Gospell about my necke, and a paire of braslettes of Corall about myne armes. Oh God,
12 defend us! I am sory that we came forthe.

Roger.

Maister and Maistres, come into this valley, and let vs sitte in that same deepe close pitte vnder the hille side untill the <small>Sodain fear.</small>
16 storme be past, Sainte George to borrowe. Mercifull God, who did euer see the like!

Ciuis.

I thinke it be the daie of iudgement; the yearth doeth quake,
20 the heauen doeth burne, and me thinke I doe see the fearfull horseman lighted in the valley with a maruelous fearfull sayng, *En adsum vobis mors vltima linia rerum, &c.* Oh, where shall we hide vs from him? He casteth forthe his .iij. dartes, and taketh them vp
24 again. He is in a greate rage; beholde how he destroieth <small>Death destroieth all creatures: none can resiste hym.</small> man and beast in this valley! This is come in a momente; who would haue thought it in the mornyng? none of us, he draweth nere; I knowe hym well, it is mercileesse
28 Death most fearfull. I am afraied of his presence; he bendeth his blacke darte against me; I haue no Target to beare it of. Alas,[1] alas! wife, wife!

Vxor.

32 Good housband, remember that I am yonge, and with childe; also you are well stricken in yerès. Therefore plaie the <small>The condition of the woman.</small> man, and take *Roger* with you, and intreate him; giue[2]

---

[1] 'Alas ... wife' omitted in ed. 1564.
[2] 'giue ... poundes' omitted in ed. 1564.

A DIALOGVE. 115

hym an hundreth poundes, and if hee will needes haue you, yet for Goddes sake be not acknowen that I am here, for feare that he kill me and your childe also.

Ciuis.

Kepe you close under that cloke, and stir not. I praie you be[1] not afraied.

Roger.

I can not abide hym. I will run awaie, for pouertie and death will part good fellowship. Sir, shift for your self, and drawe your sworde against hym. *Gentle Roger.*[1]

Ciuis.

Alas, my wife in my trouble is to fainte harted, and will not keepe me companie; my Seruaunte is runne awaie from me: whether maie I flie from death? If I doe runne, he is to swifte for me; if I tourne my backe, he will cowardlie kille me; if I dooe submitte my self to hym, he is mercilesse. I perhaps shall perswade hym with my golde; I haue an hundreth poundes in Angels. I will giue it hym to saue my life. Oh, he is heere. Sir, moste humbly here vpon my knees, I desire your lordship to pardon me, and suffer me to liue still in this worlde, and here I offer vnto you this purse of golde; I shal alwaie doe you seruice, and loue you with all my harte, and be at your lordshipes commaundement, and to my power seke to please you as my good lorde and maister. *A friende at neede.* *Death will not be entreated.*

Mors.

You are well ouertaken, I am glad that wee are mette together; I haue seen you since you were borne; I haue threatened you in all your sicknesse, but you did neuer see me nor remembred me before this daie; neither had I power to haue taken you with me vntill nowe. For I haue Commission to strike you with this blacke dart, called the pestilence; my maister hath so commaunded me; and as for gold I take no thought for it; I loue it not. No treasure can keepe me back the twinckelyng of an *Death commeth not before his time.* *Pestilence.*

---

[1] 'be not afraid' omitted in ed. 1564.
[1] In eds. 1573, 1578, this side-note is placed opposite the preceding speech.

eye from you; you are my subiect, and I am your lorde. <small>Our dales are sette.</small>
I will cut of your iourney, and separate your mariage,
but not cut of your yeeres; for thei are determined when I should
come : this is your appoincted tyme. And when the tyme shal be
appoincted me, I will smite your wife, children, and seruauntes; thei
shall not bee hidden from me. I will finde them forthe, be thei
hidden neuer so secret, or flie neuer so swift or farre of; for I am
so swifte that in a moment of an eye I can compasse the whole worlde,
and am of so wonderful a nature, that I can bee in sondrie places at
once, and in sondrie shapes. In flames of fire I often tymes doe consume mankinde; in the water I doe kill them; I am <small>What death is.</small>
marueilous in woorke. I spare nothing that hath life, but I bring
all to an ende, & to mine own nature, which is death.

Ciuis.

Sir, I moste humbly desire you too suffer me too retourne home
againe into the citie, and set my goodes in order to the vse of my
wife and children, to paie my debtes, and then godlie to departe this
worlde. I desire no more, good maister death.[1]

Mors.

I muste dispatche, and strike you with this blacke Darte; I haue
muche businesse to doe with the other twoo Dartes.

Ciuis.

Oh fearefull death, what is these twoo other Dartes in thyne
hande?

Mors.

I will smite thee with this Pestilence darte, as I haue doen to
many kingdomes, cities, and people, bothe manne and beaste, yong
and olde; with this pale darte I will destroie infinite <small>Honger.</small>
nombers, with honger thei shall perishe for lacke of foode, in destruction of corne, cattell, wine, oile, fruicte, herbe, grasse, foule, and fishe.
I will make theim eate their own fleshe, and make their <small>Greate vengeaunce.</small>
owne children to be sodden and rosted for theim. With
this thirde darte I will in battaile slaie in nomber more then the starres

---

[1] 'good maister death' omitted in ed. 1564.

of heauen, and bathe my self in bloud; I spare not one, neither
Prince nor Peasaunte, against whom I doe cast this darte. I haue
no respecte of any personc; be thei neuer so noble, riche, strong, wise,
learned, or counnyng in Physicke, thei shall neuer preuaile againste
me, but I will ouercome theim; I come into the kynges chamber at
the time appoincted, in force of Physicke, and cast my darte, that
none shall see, but feele. I often came into the comptyng house,
and sodainly killeth the money tellers;[1] I ouerthrowe the Daunser,
and stoppe the breathe of the synger, and trippe the runner in his
race; I breake wedlocke,[2] and make many widdowes; I doce sitte in
iudgment with the iudge, and vndo the life of the prisoner, and at length kille the iudge also hymself; I doe somon the greate Bishops, and cutte theim through the[3] rochettes; I vtterlie blemishe the beautie of all Courtiers, and end the miseries of the poore. I will neuer leaue till all fleshe shall bee vtterly destroied; I am the greatest crosse and scourge of God. *The greatest of all.*

Ciuis.

What is the cause, O fearfull death, that thou dooest scourge the
face of the yearth with thy dartes, and who hath sente thee for that
purpose?

Mors.

Neither is the saiyng of the Philosophers or Poetes true, whiche
compt that I come by chaunce to mortall thinges, or *Note this.*
inquiring the cause of the matter, or *Depriuatione in materia*, or of
generation and coruption; and some other do affirme that I do come
through the concorse of the starres, infecting the aire and poisonyng
liuing thinges; and therefore the Heathen in fearfull Tragidies and
Stories hath[4] admonished the vaine worlde to repente by settyng
forthe of mee Death. Some of them daiely had the dedde heddes of
their parentes broughte to their Tables, to mortifie their vanities
withall. And all these menne whom I haue slaine were Heathen
menne. But I am the messenger of God, his scourge and crosse to all
fleshe, good and badde, and am the ende of life, whiche doe separate[5]
the bodie from the soule. I am no feigned thyng by the wise

---

[1] Ed. 1564, teller.   [2] Ed. 1564, wedlockes.   [3] Ed. 1564, their.
[4] Ed. 1564, haue.   [5] Ed. 1573, separte.

braines of the Philosophers; but onelie through the disobedience of your firste Parentes, Adam and Eua, through whose fault all fleshe is corupted[1] and subiecte to mee Death; for through synne came Death.
4 Truely, my maisters anger was so greate in youre Parentes, that he suffered me to plague with my hande the beste in his Churche, as Abell, Esaie, Hier[e]mie,[2] Zacharie, John Baptiste, and Jesus Christe, his onely Sonne, whiche suffered me; and seyng that my maister
8 hath commaunded me not to spare his onely childe, with his Apostles and holy Martyres, Dooest thou thinke that I should beare with thee, or suffer any in this wicked worlde? He sent me to Sodome with his Angels, to burne them, to drouue bloudie Pharao, and
12 to slea the kinges of the Heathen; Also I was at their endes. Although al fleshe doeth abhorre me, yet Judas and all desperate men did call vpon me. Thus do I ende bothe good and badde; but precious in the sight of the lorde is the death
16 of his sainctes, and many be the scourges of wicked men. I am in Gods handes as the sworde is in the man of warres; as it is written: The Lorde doeth kill, and quicken againe, and it is he that did create euill, that is pain or death, light and darcknesse; And whereas
20 he hath not sette his strong Angel to bridle me, I am mercilesse, and will kille all whereas the token is not set vp, or his marke vpon theim whom he dooeth forbid me to touche; And that is not vpon thee nor vpon many thousandes that lieue moste
24 wretchedlie. Thy daies is but a span long; thou art like a flower in the field; thy daies are passed like a shadowe; Thou haste run thy race, and thy daies are consumed like smoke, and thou shalt scant liue to drawe thy breath. I must destroye this,
28 thy yearthly mansion, I am so commaunded: haue, here is thy rewarde, suffer it paciently. I muste goe presently to visite a greate nomber sodainly, that dooe not remember mee; I will cutte them doune with my sithe like Grasse, and kill theim with my
32 three fearfull dartes. The paines of helle doe follow me to swallowe vp al fleshe that doth not repent them of their wickednesse.

Death is horrible.

Ezech. ix.

Job xliiii.

Hell cometh after death.

---

[1] In ed. 1564 is the side-note (omitted in later eds.) 'Adam caused death.'
[2] Ed. 1564, Ieremie.

Ciuis.

Oh, wretched man that I am; whether shal I fly for succor. Now my body is past cure, no Phisicke can preuaile; Psalme 138. the sorowes of death doeth compasse me round about; the policie of the worlde with feare badde me flie, and vse Gods meanes, as Lot did when Sodome was a fire. But now doe I see who so escapeth honger and the sworde, shal be ouertaken with the pestilence; I am at the pittes brinke; nowe begin I to waxe weake in bodie; I am verie drie, my paine doeth increase, he is gone that did strike me, but I doe fele his wounde that he gaue me. Alas! woe is my vile stinckyng carcas, and filthie fleshe, conceiued and borne in sinne, depriued of original iustice, compared to a beaste in Adam, fallen as a rotten aple from a liuyng tree. What haue I gotten, my lord God, by my fall? nothing els but onely darkenesse, care, miserie, affliction, sicknesse, paine, anguishe;[1] and nowe in myne harte, death moste painfull it self now, for all my pompe, healthe, wealthe, riches, and vaine pleasures of this worlde. This my bodie, whiche I haue bothe costlie clothed, well fedde, and garnished with all delightes, for whose sake I haue been coueteous, and sinned against Jesus Christ, to maintaine the same bodie. From henceforthe, therefore, now shall I be tourned into a stinking carrion for wormes delite, duste, claie, rotten, moste vile, forsaken of all men, poore without substaunce, naked without clothyng, Sowne in dishonour, forgotten of my posteritie, not knowen from hencefoorthe, vanishe like a shadowe, wither like a leafe, and fade as a Flower. Oh! vncertaine life, but moste assured death, Fie on this filthie shadowe of this worlde, and flatteryng of the same, with all the instrumentes of the fleshe. Oh Lorde! although I[2] bee in this extreame trouble, yet haue mercie vpon me, accordyng to thy great mercie and louyng kindnesse; For I dooe make my praier in the time of trouble, trusting that thou wilt heare me.

(margin notes: No policie against death. Remember this, good reader. Man moste vile carion. 1 Cor. xv. Psalm 51 and 119.)

Roger.

Maistres, the fearfull thyng that talked with my maister is gone. Let vs goe heare what newes with hym.

[1] Ed. 1564, agues.   [2] So ed. 1564. Eds. 1573, 1578, it.

Vxor.

I am glad it is paste; thankes be to God. I will goe with speede to see my husbande, for he hath been in greate daunger.

Roger.

Sir, I am glad that he is gone; the deuill go with hym. Hath he taken all your golde?

Ciuis.

No; I haue my golde in store, for in the world I found it, and in the world I must leaue it; it is but vaine, and cannot helpe in the tyme of this my trouble. God hath preuented me, and somoned me to appeare before his seate. This Death hath smitten me: I must dye. We can carie nothyng awaia.

Vxor.

Alas! my good sweete housbande, what aileth you, Or what would you haue me do for you to helpe you in this case?

Ciuis.

Helpe me into some house, whereas I might sende for some manne of God to bee my heauenly Phisicion, teachyng me the waie to the kyngdome of Christe. The beste waie.

Roger.

Here is a house at hand, and here is your horse also; we will helpe you vp, and carrie you to this place.

Vxor.

Nowe, sir, you bee come here into this place, for Gods sake discomforte not yourself, I truste you shall dooe well; you shall want nothing that maie be had for money, gold and siluer. I will sende for your owne brethren and sisters. You shall haue with all speede the best learned Phisicions in this realme; I[1] will sende for maister doctor *Tocrub;* in the meane tyme drinke Dragon water and Mithridatum mingled together, to putte this passion from your harte. Ride, Roger! and seeke a Phisition with all speede: spare not the horse! Past remede.

---

[1] 'I ... Tocrub' omitted in ed. 1564.

Ciuis.

Softe, sirrah, and speake with me, and doe what that I dooe commaunde you, in the name of Iesus Christ.

Roger.

Sir, looke what your maistership shall commaunde me to doe, that wil I doe with all speede, and tary not.

Ciuis.

Goe thy waies, and praie maister *Theologus* to come to me, that I maie haue his counsaile; praie hym to come with speede: deliuer him this ryng.[1]

Roger.

I shall; in the meane tyme, good maister, bee of good cheare, for Gods sake.

Vxor.

Alas! what shall I dooe, and my poore children?

Ciuis.

I haue sette my wordlie thynges in order, for so hath Gods's woorde taught me to doe, I thanke God, and my debtes shall be truly paied, and whatsouer any poore man doeth owe me I doe forgiue theim, and restitution shall I make with all speede to as many as I haue wronged. And I shall leaue plentie to you and my children, requiryng you to liue accordyng to God's commaundement, obeiyng hym all the daies of your life;[2] and remember Death, and to doe to all menne as you would bee dooen vnto. To liue chaste, either in mariage or a life sole; vse praier, and chaste your bodies with abstinence. Bee pitifully mynded and hate vice, beware of wicked companie, loue well the Temple of God, visite the prisoners and helplesse; this is good Religion in the eyes of God. As nere as you can, keepe the commaundementes of almyhtie God, and beware of idlnesse and pride of harte. Lament no more, good wife, For who can kepe that must needes awaie.[3]

A wiseman.
Toby xij.
Admonition to his wife and children.

---

[1] Ed. 1564, token.   [2] Ed. 1564, liues.
[3] Ed. 1564 proceeds 'me thinke I heare Theologus come,' and then as on p. 123, 'Sir, God the heauenlie Phisicion,' &c.

Roger to hymself.

I haue spon a faire threde. I haue serued a good maister with a mischeef; he hath giuen me nothyng in his will; he is so spiritually
4 mynded that he forgetteth poore Roger, that hath taken paines for hym thes ten yeres. Well, I haue had but small gaines in seruyng hym, beyng an honest, faithfull man. What shall I doe? I will now see if I can get entertainment to liue emong knaues. I knowe
8 where a promoter dwelleth which hath muche annoyed the common wealthe. He hath gained muche, he is busie, braggyng, and shamelesse, he will despence with euery offence for money. If I misse of hym then I will go to some impudent pettie Fogger, a periured iacke
12 sauce, which can make shifte for money to the hinderraunce of many: if the worste faile [falle?], I will be a Tapster, for of all Potage I loue good Ale. I can also speake Pedlers French wel; that I can doe well with a foote packe. But now to the ende of my iourney; I will not
16 returne to my master againe, he will dye on this Plague. My Dame will haue newe Wedlocke within this sixe weekes, and as the worlde goeth now adaies, she will think it long; out of sight out of mynde.

Yet, alas, what shall I doe, poore knaue? I could goe to London,
20 and lurke in some baudie Lane. And in the nighte, when the watche is either a sleepe or gone awaie (For when the moste neede is then are the watch sonest gone), I could then, with my companions, with hookes, pick lockes, or ladders, or Gunpowder to open lockes, or
24 a Crowe of Yron make shifte for a bootie of plate, clothes, &c. But I doe fear the Gallous. I knowe an olde stale hore of myne in London; she is married to, an[1] hoddie pecke, John a Noddes. He liueth by stealyng of Horse tailes and Calfes tailes, and dooeth
28 seethe them, and sell them to the Hosiers to stop hose (because men now adaies hath smal buttockes; would God, therefore, that their hose wer greater, thei are to small). This quene will picke his purse for my sake. She can make false Dice; Hir firste housebande was
32 prentise with James Elles, and of hym learned to plaie at the shorte knife and the horne Thimble. But these Dogge trickes will bryng one to the Poxe, the Gallous, or to the Deuill. Oh, that I had as muche money as my Maister, and were a free man in London, then

---

[1] Ed. 1578, and.

would I lende my money to Vsurie, and vse false weightes and measures; and then would I plaie the Brewer, and goe into the countrie, and buie up malt as cheape as I could, and make Beere as vnprofitable to the Common wealthe for myne owne gaine; euen so 4 would I dooe in buiyng of Woode in the countrie, and causyng short Billettes to bee made, and false marke my woode when I doe sell it in London or els where. So could I make a trim hotche potche in bruyng of wine and all other wares; mingle the good with the bad, 8 as men saie, Lette the quicke Horse drawe the deade Horse out of the myre. A Dogge hath but a daie. Let the deuill paie the malt manne. Now I am nere Maister Doctour *Theologus* place, that diuine holie gentleman, he walketh in the spirite; God blesse hym. 12 I thinke as holie as he is he care not if he had twentie Benefices, thei would neuer trouble his holie conscience. Would God that I could read English trimly, I would make freendes to bee a Minister; I would learne to handle the matter well for my purpose. Well, I 16 will be sober. Howe, howe! where are you, Maister *Theologus?*

Theologus.
In the name of God, who calleth me! I am here.

Roger. 20
By your leaue, sir.

Theologus.
Welcome, good brother; what is your pleasure?

Roger. 24
Sir, my Maister and Maistresse commendeth them to your maistership. Hee is sicke; he praies you to come: here is a token.

Theologus.
God's will bee doen; I will goe with all speede. Depart with 28 speede, I will folowe.

Roger.
Fare ye well; I praie you tary not.

Theologus. 32
With all speede, good freende. Good tidynges.[1]
Sir,[2] God, the heauenlie Phisition, blesse you, and giue you the

[1] Ed. 1564, things. [2] Here ed. 1564 begins again.

perfect consolation of conscience in Christe his Sonne, and giue you grace mekely to beare this his Crosse.

Ciuis.

4 You are hartely welcome, deare *Theologus;* I have thought it longe since I did sende for you.

Theologus.

Your man declared to me by the waie a pitifull storie which 8 happened to you this daie. Further, I had soner been with you, but one Maister *Antonius* sent for me; but or I came he was dedde; and *Auarus* and *Ambodexter* is in his house preparyng a solempne Funerall for hym. _{To late.}

12 *Ciuis.*

Oh, sir, then I haue no cause to rehearse the matter newe again, but seyng my fleshe is nere the pitte, and in a manner my breath faileth me, beyng wounded with death; and that I am of twoo 16 partes, bodie and soule; the one past all cure, the other in hope of saluation; I desire, if it please God, that I may liue to the ende of your Orations. Declare vnto me what is the cause of synne.

Theologus.

20 The deuill was the first cause of synne, as it is written in Genesis, how with a lye he deceiued the woman; and thei that commit synne are of the Deuill, for he hath synned from the beginnyng of the worlde, and is the first aucthour of 24 synne. The seconde cause was man declinyng from God, credityng the Deuill, by whiche man synne entered into the world; and all the calamities and crosses therein, as sorowe, dreade, feare, pouertie, sicknesse, and Death it self, all to punishe Synne. _{Sathans worke.} _{Mannes wretchednes.}

28 *Ciuis.*

Oh, Lorde, how haue I[1] erred; I had thought God had been the cause, as when I reade these woordes, *Indurabo cor Pharonis,* I will indurate the harte of Pharao with such like places; and his indura-32 tion was the cause of his synne, and who did indurate hym but God? And when it is saied, *Ne nos inducas in tentationem,* Neither leade

---

[1] Eds. 1564, 1573, I haue.

us into temptation, &c. Here I gathered it was God that led vs into temptation, for which cause we desire hym not to lede vs into temptation, &c.

Theologus.

You haue mistaken those places, for God is not the aucthour or cause of synne, for he did so muche abhorre the same, that nothing could pacifie his wrathe under Heauen, no merite or woorke, but onelie the bloudde of Jesus Christe his Soonne; for this <small>Christes death</small> woorde I will indurate the verie woorde in Hebrue is, I wil suffer Pharoes harte to bee hardeined. And so it was in the Lordes praier, *Ne sinas nos induci,* neither suffer vs to be ledde or fall into temptation, &c. Therefore, my brother, it was the will of Sathan and man that caused synne.

Ciuis.

Why, hath not manne will to dooe good againe if he <small>Manns will.</small> luste?

Theologus.

No, if he had the election to will as first he had, he would doe the like, therefore it is in a sure hande, euen in Goddes, and not in ours; as when men doe speake the truthe, it is not of <small>Math. x.</small> their owne wil or power, but the heauenly spirite in theim. And by Almightie God are all the steppes of menne directed; though man fall into sondrie temptationes he shall not be caste of, for the Lorde putteth vnder his hand, whiche is a greate <small>Psalm xc.[1]</small> comfort to vs in trouble when wee are vnderneath the crosse. Without hym wee can dooe nothyng that is good. No <small>Jhon xi.</small> man can take any good thyng vpon hym except it be giuen to hym from heauen; and no manne, deare brother, can come to the Soonne of God vnlesse the Father hath drawen,[2] and not his will, whiche is moste wicked from his youth vpward, as appeareth in our vile nature, thought, woorde, and deede; And who soeuer <small>Roma viii.</small> hath not the spirite of Christe is not of Christe, but those whiche are ledde of the Spirite of God are the Soonnes of God; and this commeth not by mannes will and power. For the worldlie mynded

---

[1] So ed. 1564.—Ed. 1573, xxx. (cut in ed. 1578).
[2] Ed. 1564, drawen him.

manne doeth not vnderstande or perceiue thynges[1] that are of God's Spirite, without wiche it[2] can not bee saued, bee he neuer so learned and can dispute of the Soule, makyng distinc- tions of knowledge and iudgemente, callyng it the mynde or intellection, or reason, or desire, whiche is the will vnder whom the affection is gouerned, whose spryng is the harte. All these make not to the heauenlie purpose, but rather standing vpon suche trifles doeth hinder the waie to saluation in Christ, and robbe hym of his Passion when wee doe attribute freedome or freewill to come of our selues, but that we are in God's handes as his instru- mentes through hym to woorke suche thynges as beste maye please hym; and he withdrawe his holy handes, wee can doe no good, therefore submit your self to Christ and his will, for our willes are malignante and dampnable in his[3] eyes. Forsake your praue will, and submit[4] your self to Jesus Christe, sayng, now before [y]our death, Our Father whiche art in heauen, hallowed bee thy name; thy kyngdome come, Thy will be doen in yearth as it is in heauen, &c. And thus I doe conclude of freewill in vs, and faithfully to[5] looke for the rewarde, not of woorkes but of mercie onely; onely purchased by the Sacrifice of Christe; thankyng hym that he hath made you mercifull to your brethren in this world, whiche was the fruites of Faith, by which faith in his bloude wee are saued, and shall receiue our almose or rewarde, and not our duetie; for we are vnprofitable when wee haue doen our beste.

Ciuis.

What reward is that, I praie you? Or what promises are granted by Christe?

Theologus.

The reward is the remission of synnes and life euerlastyng, graunted by the father for Jesus Christes sake, freely, without our workes, for there is none other Saluation vnder heauen given vnto menne but onely Christe; in hym wee dooe

---

[1] Ed. 1564, those thynges that. [2] Ed. 1564, he. [3] Eds. 1573, 1578, our.
[4] Ed. 1564, humbly submit. [5] Ed. 1573 omits 'to.'
[6] So ed. 1578.—Eds. 1564, 1573, Jesus Christ.

merite, as when we are merciful we haue a promise of this present
life and the life to come. And in this worlde also an hundreth folde,
and in the worlde to come euerlastyng life. And who Matth. x.
that giueth one of these little ones a Cuppe of Water for my names
sake, shall not lose his rewarde. And he commaunded to giue,
promisyng it shall be giuen to them againe. And further he saieth,
Breake the breade to the poore and it shall bee to thee like a
gardein. He saieth not, let thyne Exeeutours or Assignes giue the
poore when thou art ded, but thou must doe it thy self in this
worlde, Now, while it is Light; for the night[1] is at Luke xv.
hande, I meane death, when thou canst not woorke. Remember
Diues loste the tyme, and could not call it backe againe, whiche
waileth in helle, hath no reward, for he trusted not God, nor
rewarded any man. Further, reconcile thy self to thy brother, for els
thou canst not please God, though thou[2] wroughtest all good workes,
and gaue thy bodie to be burned; for Charitie is so 1 Cor xiii.
precious in Gods eyen, that who so wante it cannot reigne with
Christ; Therefore, forgiue from thy hart and thou shalte be forgiuen.
Make not thy will vpon goodes gotten by Vsurie, nor by any thing
falsely[3] in bargainyng thou hast taken from thy brother, Psalme xiiii.
for then thou shalt not dwell in gods tabernacle, neither shall thy
children prosper upon the yearth, but God will hate theim to the
thirde and fowerth generation, for thy synne. Examine Psalme liii
well thy conscience. Death hath wounded thee, whiche is common
to all fleshe: in thus doyng thou shalt passe from Death to euerlastyng life by Christ, And neuer taste vpon the seconde death emong
the impious or caste awaies. Confesse thy synnes from thy harte;
aske mercie, bee thei neuer so red and many in number; Psalme lj.
Jesus hath washed them in his bloud, and sprinckled them with
Hysope, and made theim as white as Snowe. Now plaie the manne
in Christe; feare not to departe this worlde; Christe is gone before
with his holie Prophetes,[4] Apostles, Martyres, Confessours, and Virgins,
penitent theeues, and harlottes, also there is the Armie of Angelles
before his Throne, with ioye incessantly honouryng hym. Hell

---

[1] Eds. 1573, 1578, light.   [2] Ed. 1578, ye.
[3] Ed. 1564, thing that falsly.   [4] Ed. 1564, Apostles, Prophetes.

gates are sparred, Sathan beaten doune, thy synnes rased, <small>Apoc. vltimo.</small>
the good Angell at hande to conducte thee to that blessed lande
of rest; here is nothyng but labour, daies of care, synne, wretchednesse, a thousande crosses, the snares of the deuil, and many vanities,
the fleshe moste inconstaunte, the worlde a place of miserie and
synne: bidde it farewell, takyng thy leaue with the badge <small>Christian mans badge.</small>
of a Christian manne of Christe crucified; remember
that promise made in thy Baptisme. Arme thy self with the breast
plate of faithe, continue to the ende, And thou shalt receiue a
crowne of life; thy crosse taken awaie, cast thy whole <small>2 Cor. xv.</small>
care vppon Christe, and he shall deliuer thee at hande, and giue
thee the holy Resurrection of bodie and soule to dwell in one for
euer with hym.

Ciuis.

Oh, what comforte in conscience I haue receiued. First, I
render thankes to God the Father, the Soonne, and the <small>Comforte in conscience.</small>
Holie Ghoste. Secondlie, blessed bee the hower of
youre commyng hether in this time[1] of my trouble with this holie
consolation in Christe, in whom I dooe beleue, renounsyng the
worlde, the fleshe, and the deuill; beleuyng all the Articles of my
Christian faithe, acknowledgyng the blessed Sacramentes <small>Sacramentes.</small>
to bee the instrumentes to euerlastyng life, And saluation in Christ,
by the whiche God doeth woorke in his Churche to the worldes ende,
to them that shall bee saued; one Trinitie, and three distincte
persones, coequall in vnitie, in one essence and beyng is <small>The holie trinitie.</small>
my God: the Father created me, the Sonne redeemed me,
and the Holie Ghost sanctified me and inspired me, whereby I
knowe that I am his elected; and one vndefiled mother, the churche,
hath thus taught me in that blessed booke of Patriarkes, Prophetes,
Martyres, and Jesus with his Apostles, which is Goddes woorke.
Now, Maister Theologus, my tyme is at hande; I praie you saie
some thyng of the Resurrection, and then let vs praie in the name
of God together, that it maie please hym to forgiue me <small>The holie churche.</small>
my synnes, whiche I have committed against heauen
and yearth, and to receiue my Soule into his blessed handes.

---

[1] Eds. 1573, 1578, into the time.

Theologus.

Good brother, not onely the doctrine of Prophetes and the Euangelistes doe promise the Resurrection to come, of some to saluation, and some to dampnation, but the same Resur- Matth. xxvii. rection is most manifeste. As, for example, Christe hymself and other did rise, and were seen to many in Hierusalem; and by the space of fourtie daies he taughte the Apostles, and was conuersaunte with theim, and then ascended into glorie, vntil the Matth. xiii. tyme appointed to judge the quicke and the dedde, when he shall sende his Angelles to gather all fleshe vnder heauen from the fower Windes, and sitte doune to Judgement, saiyng, Come to me, you blessed of my[1] Father, and receiue the kyngdome prepared for you from the beginnyng. Further he saith, this is the wiil of my father whiche hath sent me, that all that doe see the Soone, and beleue[2] in him, shall haue euerlasting life, and I will raise hym in the last daie. And the holie Apostle Sainct Paule moste heauenly doeth preach the resurrection to the Corinthians. The[3] dead shall liue, saieth Esai, and thy slaine shall rise againe.; and thei[4] Esaie lviii. whiche slepe in the duste shall rise; the yearth shall cast forthe their dead bodies. I will create bothe Heauen and Yearth newe, saieth the Lorde, and putte the old out of my remembraunce. Many, saith Daniel, that lye a slepe in the dust shalbe Daniel xii. wakened againe, some to life euerlastyng, and other to reprobation. God saieth, I will open their tombes, and bryng them Math. xxv. forthe. And the holie man Job saieth, I knowe that Job xix. my Redemer liueth, and that in the last daie he shall raise me again out of the yearth, and shall be clothed again with my skin, and in my fleshe. I shall se God, whom I shall se with these[5] same eyes, and with none other. These are comfortable and most true places of holie Scripture for the resurrection of the dead. You are assured in conscience of this blessed resurrection and life euerlasting in Christ Jesus our Lorde.

Ciuis.

Yea, forsouthe, deare *Theologus*, but my speache is almoste paste,

[1] Ed. 1564, the. [2] Ed. 1564, beleueth. [3] Ed. 1564, Thy.
[4] Ed. 1564, those. [5] So ed. 1564.—Eds. 1573, 1578, the.

yet I thank God I know you all, and I beseche him to blesse you, and when my Spirite is gone, I praie you burie my bodie with comelinesse, not with pompe, and vse it as an instrumente wherein the Soule hath dwelled, and whiche the Soule shall possesse again in honour in that blessed Resurrection.

Theologus.

Lette vs moste humblie, here upon our knees, with our handes lifted vp towardes the heauen, desire God the Father, for Christes sake, to receiue your Soule into his glorious kyngdome. *Exhortation to death.*

O, deare citezen, reioyce and be glad that thy labour is almoste past; rest is at hande; feare not the Paine of Death, For it is impossible to escape that which can not bee fledde or auoided. For it is written, who is that man that liueth and shal not see death? none; no, not one. Therefore suffer it, my swete harte, paciently; and that is an argument of good conscience, and of an heauenly mynde. Youre wife mourneth immoderately. Oh God, all fleshe was borne to dye. This happened to our *All flesh shall[1] dye.* parentes, as father, mother, &c., And shall not faile to all that shall followe vnto the ende of the woorlde, or commyng of Christe. For surely sweete life was neuer withont the exception of bitter death; it is no noueltie; therefore, when we dooe heare tell of the departure of anie of our frendes, let vs not fall into a sodaine passion, as one Ely the high priest did, whiche hearyng of the death of his children, felle doune and brake his necke: but rather constantly with wise Anaxagoras, which hearyng of the death of his beloued sonne, saied to the messenger, this is no newe tidynges, nor strange to me; as sone as he was borne, I knewe that he should die, for of Natures lawe is learned life to be taken and resigned, and no man dye but he which hath liued. Oh, leaue your lamentyng, good maistres; why rage ye like one whiche haue no hope? Be absent, or vse moderation; remember holie Job, the same daies when the lord permitted Sathan not onely to destroy his seruants and cattell, but also, before age, in the lustie tyme of youth, in the feast daie, at one table, his deare children *A constant wiseman in adversitie.* *Of Jobes pacience.*

[1] Omitted in eds. 1573, 1578.

of his bodie were all broken in peeces and slaine with the violent fall of the house. What, did he rende his heare or fleshe? no, no; he considered who sent them, and who did take them; euen the lorde, whom he moste obediently suffered, and reuerently thanked. Further, good sister, remember Saincte Hierome takyng God too witnesse of an holie woman whose husbande was dedde, whom she[1] moste tenderly loued, by whom she had but twoo Sonnes of singular beautie, wantyng no gifte of grace, or of nature, whiche bothe died the same daie wherein their father departed. When this Crosse was, saieth S. Hierome, who would not haue thoughte that she woulde haue fallen madde in rendyng her heare, breastes, clothes, and skin, running vp and doune, wailyng and cryng with pitiful wryngyng of handes? What did she? First she weped not one teare, but moste soberly, with a womanly countenance, she humbly kneled upon her knes, holdyng up her handes, rendering thankes, and makyng praiers to Almightie God, sayng, Most humblie I thanke thee, good Lorde, for that that it hath pleased thee to take me into thy seruice; I am sped, Oh Lorde, for thou haste discharged me, &c. Take also for an example the moste worthie constance[2] of that paciente woman, whiche, without muche lamentation, did with her own eyen beholde her deare children slaine, their members cutte in peces and boiled in Caldrens. Marke how constauntly of late yeres children did see the fleshe of their fathers, mothers, &c., burne in the fire moste pacientlie sufferyng; And, againe, fathers beholdyng their children dooe the like. What, did thei roare like Lyons, &c.? No, no; but reioysed that God had of their bloud and stocke erected a people to reigne with hym in life, whiche witnessed him in death. The examples should moue all Christians perfecte, mortification is not. muche to lamente for our frendes diyng, but rather by the example of their deathes to remember our ende, and then wee shall not synne. Therefore, better it is to goe to the house of mournyng then to the house of banquettyng; and when it shall please God to call your housebande awaie, and the daies of forgetfulnesse shall approche, as euery thing vnder heauen haue the tyme bothe of mournyng and reioysyng.

A constant woman in trouble.

Counsaile: A blessed woman, 2 Macha. vii.

Remember our ende.

[1] Ed. 1564, he.   [2] Ed. 1564, constauncie.

When you doe beholde your self in a glasse, remember *A glasse.*
your face shall bee leane and pale, your nose rotten, your tethe
stinkyng and blacke, your eyen dimme and blinde, your eares deafe,
and runnyng, your Heeres fallen awaie, your Vaines broken, your
Senewes relaxed, and wasted, bones corupted, bowels ful of roumes,
and all your fleshe consumed. Beholde, beholde, you damosels of
vanities, and lustie youth, the pleasure of this worlde, *A glasse for faire gentle-*
how it endeth with stinke, filthe, &c., not reserued after *women.*
death to any good purpose, as timber when it is cutte doune, but
because it is so vile and will infecte the ayre, The corps inclosed[1]
in a pitte, as we daiely see, whereas it consumeth, as I haue saied.
Remember this; be not proude of noble parentage, of riches, beautie,
or cunyng, but rather consider where are the old lustie *Where are the old noble*
Kynges, Queenes, Lordes, Knightes, Ladies? Where are *persons?*
the old courtiers, and valiaunt men of warre? Where are the Maiors
of cities, Lawiers, Bishoppes, Phisicions? Where are all the pleausante
Musicions? Where are become the olde Commons in euery Kyngdome?
Where is become the Popes rotten holinesse, with all the infernall
malignaunte Synagoge of Antichriste, &c.? All are gone and passed
like shadowes, wasted, and come to nothing, as Saincte Augustine
affirmeth. Oh man, saieth he, goe to the cha[r]nell house *De van. hujus mundi.*
or graues, take vp the bones, marke well if thou canst *The greatest of*
knowe the master from the seruaunt, the faire from the *the dedde.*
foule, the riche from the poore, the wise from the foole, &c. Thou
canste not dooe it; it is impossible to knowe theim. Well, worlde,
well, what dooest thou promise vnto all theim whiche doe loue thee?
perhaps muche riches or dignite. How noisome to the *The burden of*
soule is riches; the verie minister of, or to, all euill[2] rule *riches.*
and mischief, as damnable Vsurie, Adulterie, Treason, Murther; it
maketh one proude, high minded, and forgetfull of hymself. It
deludeth hym with flatterers and curtesies of Hypocrisie, it is the
mother of vaunglorie, and nourisher of Pride and idle life, and
lothlie glottonie. It is remembered by our Maister Jesus Christe,
whiche calleth it thornes, and by his Apostles, whiche nameth it
the roote of al euill. It is the maister of some riche men and

---

[1] Ed. 1564, is enclosed.   [2] Ed. 1578, ciuill.

women, whiche kepeth it too their greate hurte. And the foolishe Prodigall waster, whiche commonlie succedeth the gatherer, spendeth it sone awaie in wickednesse, as it is saied, easie gotten gooddes are sone spente. Therefore, sufficient, or a meane, is well to a Christen man for sundrie causes. For thei that will be riche fall into sondrie temptations, cares, broken sleapes. He gapeth and looketh for muche, and spendeth little; hee can not bee merie for feare of losse. The more he getteth he is neuer satisfied; that is a coueteous man, but still desiereth, and neuer pacified, like vnto the drie man in a hotte burning Feuer. Riches hath poisoned the churche, and transformed the Cleargie, specially in Roame, emong the Popes, and many greate men, whose auncestours[1] did keepe plentifull houses of the one halfe, whiche nowe is come too passe that nowe a daies in kepyng hospitalitie, or mynisteryng of charite, but breake vp houses, and hurt manie poore, euen for the loue of one glotton hymself, which will not well spende it, nor for his children, whiche can not well vse riches. For we doe see how God doeth plague the sede of extorcioners, vile vsurers, &c. What if thei had mountaines of golde, so increased dolour of mynde, and death stealeth on all fleshe like a theefe, and smiteth the money louer, the Vsurer, the Oppressour, the golden watchman, the greate officer, marchaunt, the wise gentleman, that hath purchased so muche. What is the ende of this geare? a dedde carkesse and scant a good windyng shete: out of the doore he must too graue; he shall farewell *Gloria mundi*, and welcome silie Wormes. I praie God that this tourneth not to dampnation. Oh, what is become of riche *Segnior Antonius* treasures?[2] *Capax, Rapax, Tenax, Ambodexter* (euill gotten goodes are worse spente), Sower sweetenesse and slippyng ise, The golden intangled hooke, and the drinke of Midas hath vtterly destroied hym, and, or euer he was aware, death hath slaine hym. He loued so well this worlde, and life in the same, that if his[4] Phisicion might haue saued his life he would haue loste one of his handes, and suffered his fleshe to haue been cut, with some broken

Sidenotes: Spendeall succeedyng Gathrall. Coueteous menne still couet. Riches helpe not in the day of vengeance. What paines men[3] will suffer to flie death.

---

[1] Ed. 1564, auncitours. [2] Ed. 1564, treasurers.
[3] Ed. 1564, man. [4] Ed. 1578, this.

bones, with the continuance of paine, ache, and griefe, with dreadfull slepes; and when he did see no remedie, the terrour of conscience tormented hym, vexed hym, and ouercame hym, made him rage and curse the tyme of his birthe; his life was so horrible in the eyes of God and man; whose iudgement I doe commende to God, but surely greate plagues doe remaine for the vngodlie. Therefore, let vs bee conuerted, and tourne cleane from our synnes and wickednesse, and so there shall no synne dooe vs harme. Lette us faste and praie, hate euill, and cleaue to good, make restitution, forgiue our enemies, abhorre vice, and be sorie that we can not be sorier. Remember our accomptes, and come betimes vnto the Lorde; make no tarryng too tourne vnto the Lorde; put not of from daie to daie. For sodainly shall his wrathe come, and in tyme of vengeance shall he destroy vs, and excepte wee doe all repent we shall perishe, saieth Christ. Let vs repent, therefore, and tourne vnto God, that he may forgiue vs, that our synnes maie bee dooen awaie, that we maie saie, From Plague, Pestilence, and Famine, from battaile and murther, and from sodaine death, Oh Lorde, deliuer us. From hardnesse of harte, and contempte of thy woorde and commaundment, whiche is the greateste cause of the wrathe and indignation, Oh good Lorde, deliuer thy people, for thy holie name sake. Amen. Amen.

Forgiue enemies.

Sodinlie cometh vengaunce.

A[1] praier in the tyme of death.

Almightie and moste deare Father of heauen, wee moste humblie beseche thee, for Jesus[2] Christe sake, haue mercie vpon this thy seruaunt, which now is nailed to the painfull crosse of death for Adams offence. Impute no synne vnto this penitent, whiche moste willingly[3] hath submitted hymself to thy fatherly correction; but behold thy sonne on the right hande, the onely Mediatoure for all the elected, whose names are written in the booke of life. Let this thy seruaunt, we beseche thee, moste mightie God, haue cleane remission and forgiuenesse of all his sinne, by thought, woorde, and deede, committed against thy diuine Maiestie; now in this perill of death, assiste hym with thy holie Aungell,

Hebr. xi.

The best medicen.

---

[1] Ed. 1564 (where the words stand as a side-note), "A praier in trouble or death."   [2] Ed. 1564, Jesus sake.   [3] Ed. 1564, willing.

commaunde Sathan to departe, make cleane his conscience, with a glad minde to reioice onely in thy mercie, for vaine is the helpe of man; but thy mercie doeth endure for euer; we are thy people, and the shepe of thy pasture: to thee we shall giue praise, for euer and euer. Amen.

Ciuis.

Amen, Amen. Lorde, receiue my soul into thy handes, thou God of truth. *A blessed ende.*

Theologus.

The almighty[1] God of Angelles, and the former of all thynges visible and vnuisible,[2] in whose handes is onely life & death, light and darknesse, and all the motions of the soule and bodie; without the, moste mightie God, all things had been nothyng, and of nothyng all thinges are made by thee; without thee,[3] Christe and thy blessed Spirite, whiche is one coeternall Trinitie, all fleshe were accursed, all consciences molested, and al soules vtterly dampned, From light into darknesse, from freedome into euerlastyng reprobation. But by Jesus Christe, thyne onely Sonne, wee thanke thee, deare father of all mercie, that nowe it hath pleased thee to take to thy mercie at this present tyme our brother, whom thou hast elected, consecrated; and now he shall by thy mercie and pitte be sanctified vnto thee to bee a Citezen of eternall glorie, now dooe fleshe and bloudde forsake hym, and all his worldlie strength faileth hym. Now is the Orgaines yeldyng up the heauenly sounde, his soule

A praier in the tyme of death.

Through the holy Trinitie is creacion & saluacion.

commeth nowe vnto thee, good Lorde; receiue it to
thy mercie, into thyne euerlasting glorie, where
as Abraham, Isaac, and Iacob are: continually to thee, oh heauenlie father,
be incessaunte honour
and glorie. Amen.

The ende of the
Dialogue.

---

[1] Ed. 1564, mightie.   [2] Ed. 1564, inuisible.   [3] Ed. 1564, thy Christ.

A copie of a letter to Frances Barlow by W. B.

When the tyme of trouble draweth nere (good Frances Barlowe),
as Death, whiche shall separate the soule from the bodie; if we bee not ware, and wisely prouidente, wee shall stande in greate daunger of losses; first we shall lose our health, strength, and beautie, wherein wee haue delighted; and all our senses, *Vanitie, plaine vanite in this worlde.*
as pleasure of speache, ioye of harte, and the comfortable sighte of the eyes, wherewith we dooe daiely beholde all the pleasures of this worlde, &c. Wee shall lose all our further treasures, landes, and substaunce, and also our liues, and as dunge bee cast into the yearth, and finallie, our soules banished from Goddes blessed presence or restyng place. Therefore let vs call, my Frances, to our remembraunce the fearefull curses of almightie God againste our synnes, and the cause of our plagues, whiche is our abhominable liuyng in synnyng againste God, in thought, woorde, and deede, againste heauen and yearth; in pride, wrathe, Idolatrie, fornication, swearyng, luste, glottonie, and stoppyng our eares againste grace and the woorde of truthe. Lette vs call to remembraunce how that we haue doen wrong to eche other in woorde and deede, in slaunderyng, or[1] hinderyng, by bargainyng, &c., our brethren for whom Christ hath died; whom wee haue hated, and not pitied in their extreame sorowes and aduersities, and haue not paied their labours *Restitution.*
and trauailes; lette vs repente and call for grace, and restore now while we are in the waie of grace, and in that that wee cannot make satisfaction for our synnes by no merites of almose, praiers, oblations, &c., whiche are vncleane in Gods eyes, as concernyng the remission of our synnes; as Job saieth: Howe can he bee cleane *Job xxiij.* that is borne of a woman? Beholde he wil giue no light vnto the Moone, and the Starres are vncleane in his sight; how muche more man, a worme, euen the Sonne of manne,[2] whiche is but a worme, whiche in beholdyng of his synne, hath no cause but to dispaire and to bee dampned. What remedie in this case? None, but with all speede, by faithe, lifte vp our hedde, and beholde euen Jesus Christe

---
[1] Ed. 1564, or in.   [2] Ed. 1564, of a man.

on Gods right hande, pleading our case, excusing vs to his father, whiche praieth to hym for vs; and is hearde, and Sathan beaten doune, and Gods Angell set at our bedside with spirituall armour for vs, in this battail of death against Sathan, to conducte vs to that happie lande; let vs kneele doune, and first saie, whatsoeuer God dooeth sende to vs, life or death, his name be praised; Gods will. his will be doen in yearth as it is with his Angels in heauen, desyring hym to bee fedde with his liuelie woorde and blessed Sacramente, the immortal foode for the soule, passing al worldly treasures or Phisicke for the bodie, and that it would please hym to pardone our trespasses and offences, in thought, worde, and deede, against his diuine Maiestie, euen as wee doe forgiue our enemies suche faultes as thei dooe here in yearth againste vs; and that in the tyme of agonie, or paines of death, he suffer vs not to fall into temptation or be ouerladen vnder our crosse, But that his hande maie help vs, and deliuer vs from this vile life, full of miseries, and bryng vs into the land of the liuing. In doyng this The lande of you shalbe moste happie and blessed; let vs submit our the liuyng. selues to hym that hath made vs: wee haue not made our selues; wee are his vessels, and are in his sight, and cannot flie[1] Genesis ii. from his presence nor run beyonde that rase whiche he Sapien. x. hath appoincted us; he bringeth Death, and restoreth Math. xxv. againe to life in the resurrection. Oh! be contented[3] to render the same talent, whiche was but lent vnto you, euen your bodie, the giftes of nature and grace: Committe wife, children, and all to hym. He dooeth no wrong: he taketh but his owne. Yelde all to God. Remember he brought you in hether naked, and how Job xiiii. you dooe liue but a small tyme, and are full of miserie; Like a flower for the tyme, and shall passe awaie like a shadowe. Alas, wee dooe deserue greate punishment, but he plageth vs not accordyng to the grauitie of our synnes, for then were wee dampned, or like vnto Sodome, that perished without handes in Lamen. iii. the daie of Gods wrath and vengaunce. Consider, Frances, that this is no newes or marueilous chaunce that you should change your life; well, it happened to all our forefathers, from Adam to

---

[1] Ed. 1564, flee. [2] Ed. 1564, Job xiii. [3] Ed. 1564, content.

kynges, and all the nobles of the yearth, and to the poore also. All fleshe is grasse, and the[1] wormes are the companions to the corps, in darke graue or house of claie. <small>All fleshe is grasse.</small>

4 Yet there is a daie whiche God hath appoincted, whiche none can tell but hymself,[2] in whiche he will iudge bothe the quicke and dedde, and call all fleshe before hym. Bothe his verie electe and the mercilesse reprobates, and then bodie and soule shall remaine 8 immortall together, and haue life euerlastyng. This holde faste, deare Frances, as an anker in this storme from death to life euerlastyng. Holde faste the twelue articles of the Christian faithe; Praie to the ende, onely to God the father, by Christ; remember 12 his promises, that at what tyme soeuer a synner doeth repente, he will forgiue; Call, he will aunswer vnto thy soule; <small>Eccl. xi.</small> knocke, and he will open. This tyme of your aduersite, and plague of the Pestilence, doeth make you forget all pleasures and delites 16 paste; euen so remember this worlde is the more slipperie, and the pleasures doe compasse all vnderstandyng to Gods elected. Because I will conclude, the tyme draweth at hande of oure deliueraunce; caste your care onely vpon God almightie, looke not backe againe, 20 beware of by pathes, either vppon the righte or lefte hande, but treade in the true pathe or verie waie of Jesus Christe hymself. I praie you let Ambrose Barnes rede the xi Chapter of sainct Ihons Gospell, and the firste Epistle to the Corinthians, the xv Chapiter.[3] 24 If the tyme had not been so muche spent, and the venime so daungerous, and the partes[4] so weake and feble, I would haue caused you to be letten bloud, and giuen you pilles *contra pestem*, with cordials accordyngly, by Gods grace, if that would haue doen you any 28 good: but take this cordial in good part. Thus God giue you the Croune of life, whiche Jesus Christe, without our deseruynges, hath purchased for vs in his precious bloud: His name bee praised. Amen.

Your W. B.

32   Fare ye well. We must followe
          when it pleaseth God.

FINIS.

---

[1] Ed. 1564 omits 'the.'
[2] Eds. 1564, 1573, have here a marginal note: 'Matth. xviij (1573, xxv); Luke xix.'   [3] Ed. 1564, chapiter xv.   [4] Ed. 1564, parties.

To[1] *his louyng frende and brother, M.*
Willyam Conscience, Minister,
W. B. sendeth salutacion.

If the almightie God do take care for the foules of the aire and flowers of the fielde, and prouideth nourishement for them, Luke xii. Math. v. how much more for his beloued men that do faithfully serue him in the holy ministerie of his worde and sacramentes, visiting the sicke and buriyng the dedde? The capitaine that doeth but seruo a mortal Prince, how so euer he spedeth, life or death, behauing himself wisely and valiauntly against the enemie, is worthy of worldly fame and honor; moche more the Lordes armoured knight, beyng Gods messenger. Mala. i. his Aungel and mouth, betwene him and his people that stande in daunger, is worthie in Christe to bee noumbred, crouned and placed among his Aungelles immortall: by this I knowe that you are no hireling, but (under Christe) the true Shepeherde, in that that you flie not from youre folde when that Wolfe Sathan with his companion Death doce woorke their violence against the flesh & soule. In this case remember these wordes: *Nolite eos timere qui occi-* Ihon. x. *dunt corpus,* &c. Feare not them whiche doe kill the bodie, thei can not kill the soule. In this we dooe see what the power of death is, onely[2] to kille in us the fower Elementes whereof the bodie is framed (by sworde, fire, water, sicknes, &c.). But the soule is not made of any of theim, but the Creatour of al thing hath made it moste pure of nothing, vpon which soule death hath no power, because it is of nature immortall. But so long as bodie and soule are together & August. de spiritu & anima. not deuided, that is called manne. And whatsoeuer thinges Cap. xliii. &c. are seen with bodily iyen are ordeined for the same bodie, and the bodie for the soule, and the soule for God. The life of the bodie is the soule, and the life of the soule is God: so for synne the bodie is ruinated and shalbe in dust until the resurrection. But in the fal or death of the bodie the soule dieth not but is deliuered, when the snare of this flesh is broked. The fleshe with the sences are dedde, Psal. cxxiiii. but *Anima cum ratione sua* doe still liue: therefore I trust The soule dieth not. and knowe that you doe consider wisely thre thinges. The first is, the world with the wretchednesse therein worthy to bee despised.

[1] These epistles and the *Table* are found only in ed. 1564.
[2] Ed. 1564, *not* onely.

The second, our owne knowledge of our selues, our synne, our sicknesse, and whereof wee are made, even of repugnaunte eelementes. Thirdly, is to laie hande of eternall blessednesse, remembring the mercifull promises of God: As come to me all you that are Matt. xii. heauie laden either with affliction of minde, pouertie in Christ, sicknesse or death, and I shall refreshe you. This is the verie Phi- The best Phisicion of the soule, even Christe, and the perfit quietnesse sicke. of conscience. God hath geuen you a talent full godlie, you doe lucretie the same and hide it not. Therefore it shalbee said moste ioyfully: it is well dooen good seruaunt and faithfull, thou haste been faithfull in little, I will make thee ruler ouer moche, enter Matt. xxv. into thy maisters ioie. And againe, he whiche doth continue to thende shall haue the croune of life. Bee paciente, my brother James v. (Conscience) and settle your harte, for the commynge of the Lorde draweth nere, and blessed are the dedde which dye in the Lorde, for thei shall reigne with Christe in glory, his name be euer praised; and his will be fulfilled. Amen. Be of
good comforte, and caste awaye
feare: be merie, let not the
Pestilent corses nor
the noyse of
belles ter-
rifie
you.

Inter mortales te non mihi charior vllus:
Te plus quam verum diligo amoque fratrem.

Finis.

COLENDISSIMO FRA-

TRI SUO IN CHRISTO, MAGISTRO

Richardo Turnero Theologo,

Gulielmus Bullenus.

S. P. D.

*Reuerendissime & obser-*uandissime frater, puto te literas meas recepisse, in quibus tibi scribebam regimen contra pestem, ac idcirco modo non ero prolixior in febre pestilenti. Nam omnis febris quam pestilentem vocamus prouenit e putredine quae sit ab excessu[1] humidi. Ha[n]c vero (ut inquit *Causa pestis.* Galenus) febrem ex plurima humiditate putrefacta prouenire putrefacta[m] sine dubio potius quam a calore aucto fatendum est. Humiditas ideo materia est putrescens in venis unde calor naturalis *Signa pestis.* valde efficitur & uno die omnes virtutes decidunt, urinae sunt fœtentes, &c. Galenus, Auic., Rasis, Trallianus, &c. affirmant: in febre pestilenti est multitudo obstructionum et praecipue ubi materia urget ad cutim & caput. Multitudo materiae et cruditatum in causa est.

Cura est prohibere putredinem. Obstructiones igitur sunt aperiendae. Sed si natura movit tunc nihil movendum est. Hoc est autem remedium, ut inquit Johannes Baptist. Monta. Viro- *Curatio in quam considerandum.* nensis: ℞ Syrup de Cichorio cum Rhabarbaro ʒ 1. ss., aqua Boraginis, acetosae ʒ 3 in quibus citrum sit impositum & decoctum deinde vnguentum pectorale contra pestem, ℞ vnguenti Rosacei confortatiui mesues ʒ j., specierum cordialium ʒ j. Sandalorum alborum ℈ j. Rosarum siccarum ʒ ss. misce simul artificiose & fiat linimentum pro corde & pro toto [*sic*] regione ventris. Mirum est hoc remedium *Dieta in tem-porae* [sic] *pestis.* contra venenum pestis. Quod ad rationem victus attinet, ubi est maxima putredo (ut inquit. Hyppo. 17. Aphoris.), ubi corrupti humores & putridi, nihil perniciosius quam instituere tenuem victum quia inter exhibeas ius pulli & ponas semper in tuo cibo preter acetosam [*sic*] succum citri. De reliquo velim tibi persuadeas quemadmodum legisti in Galeno, &c. Vale & vale iterum (eruditiss. vir) sis que; bono animo. Nunc literas concludo. Nam plura non opus habeo scribere, ne tuis optimis occupationibus (in vinea domini) importune nunc obstrepere videar. Martii Incarnati. 1564.

Tuus ad omnia Guil. Bullenus.

---

[1] Ed. 1564, excessum.

AMANTISSIMO AC PRO-
bissimo viro magistro T. Gaylo,
Chyrurgo. Guilihelmus
Bullenus. S. P. D.

BOnam valetudinem cum corporis tum animi a deo opt. max. tibi precor (optime vir). Nihil est hoc tempore quod tibi scribam quàm quòd libellum quem mihi donasti legi et iterum legi, quo tibi ago gratias & habeo ut pro sunno [sic] *munere. Nam ex eo & intellexi amorem et animum quem erga me geris, & operam tuam perspexi non solum mihi sed omnibus qui ubique sunt Anglis futuram utilitati. Nostrum enim omnium haberi possunt amatores & cultores libri tui insignissimi. Quamobrem quid magis mihi gratum esse potuit hoc munere, praesertim cum a tali Chirurgo mihi datum sit? cujus rei nunquam me capiet oblivio, sed quantum potero gratias referri libenti animo faciam. Opto te bene valere ac interim me tibi comendo; doctissimo viro magistro Bactero humillime*
meis verbis gratias agi
meque plurimum co-
mendare desi-
dero.

Martii 28. Anno incarnati
1564.

Tibi deditissimus
Guilihelmus Bu.

The Table of this presente booke.

A poore manne seking relief [1]	Page 5	A lande where as no sicknesse is	26
A wives answer to the poore man	idem	America	idem
A tale of the poore manne against couetousnes	6, 7, 8, 9	A dreadfull case	idem
		A troubled conscience	27
Antonius Capistranus the riche man	9	A Pothicaries repentaunce	idem
		A tyme to purge	idem
Antonius the Phisician	idem	A yerely reward	29
A subtile marchaunt man	11	A greate losse	idem
Antonies aungelles	12	A knavishe lackey	idem
A swete texte	idem	A mule loste	idem
A medler with no scripture	idem	*Aristotle de coelo & mundo*	31
A good indifferent man	13	A description of the soule	32
An infidell	14	Actus, what it is	34
A man of good religion	idem	Adversitee	35
A papist, a protestant	idem	*Aetuis de rei medicae*	36
A nulla fidian	idem	Avicen noteth of the pestil.	idem
A fine garden	idem	Anticedent of the pestilence	idem
A piller in a garden	15	Aire infected	idem
Antonies armes	idem	Avicens counsaill	40
A good observacion	idem	A pouder for the plague	42
An exclamation of Skelton	16	A drinke for the pestilence	idem
A saiyng of Chaucer	17	A perfume for the pestilence	43
An admonishion of Lidgat	idem	A medicen for a carbuncle	47, 48
A young Courtier	idem	A caviat for a Chyrurgian	46
A saiyng of sir Davie Linse to Englande and Scotland	18	A lotion for a sore	47
		A medicen for a plage sore	idem
A saiyng of the Phisicion	19	A Cicatrice moste best	48
Avarus a pettie fogger	idem	A healyng oyntment	idem
Ambo dexter	20	A Cordiall	55
A blacke Sainctus	idem	An Epicures talke	50
Ambo dexter gapeth for Antonius death	21	A horsewoman	58
		A nise cockney of London	59
A maiden in Antonius house	22	A churle incarnate	70
A simple practise	idem	A tale of Foxes	70
A craftie villaine	23	An epitaph of a covetous	71
A cousin made	idem	A young man well nurtred	80
A periurer	idem	A parler with many things	80
A serpent	24	A taker, a catcher	82
A good companie	25	A wicked iudge	84

[1] Fol. in Ed. 1564. The figures have been altered to agree with the present Edition.

THE TABLE.

Note adversitee	85
A lesson for a lubbar	91
A wretche which refused good counsail	90
A ruffen	95
Amber grice	99
A greate losse to England	100
A good common wealth	105, 110
A swymmyng lande	101
A praier in death	134
A letter to maister Willyam Aileward called Conscience	139
A letter to maister Richard Turner of Canterburie	141
A letter to maister Thomas Gaile Chyrurgian	142

B
Beastes did speake	page 61
Borders in a cloth	89
Barnit fielde	60
Byrdes of straunge shapes	99
Bankruptes	90

C
Clisters	27
Closenes in usury	70
Children sicke of the mother	83
Cruell women	100
Christes death	126
Carbo & antrax	45
Causes of the pestilence	36

D
Dogges and women	61
Death killeth } Death worketh } Death horrible }	pp. 118, 119
Death wil not be intreated	115
Death, what it is	116
Death endeth all	119
Death destroieth all	114
Death apereth with three dartes	idem

F
Flatterers of noble men	86
Faire fieldes	112
Feare and dred	113
Fre will in man	126

G
Gloses	25
God	32
Golden raake	82
Good ayre	39
Good observations	43
Gentle Roger	62
Galen ad Pisonem	39
Gentleman, what he is	110
Galen de diffe. feb.	36

H
Honest landlordes	112
His wiues councell	56, 57
Honger	116
Hosteler	80

I
Ingratitude	64
Iacke Drake	64
Ionge Renob	69
Iacke a napes played at tables	99
Ionge and folishe	90

K
Knavery	67

M
Mony doth great mischief	84
Mulier a naughty worde	81
Many usurers	72
Magus and Iudas	83
Makeshiftes	90
Mendax is described	94
Mendax kinred & armes	96
Mendax hath been in florida	idem
Mendax bringeth good newes	98
Mixed bodies	31

N
Newes from Florida	96
No winde but turne some to profite	9
Note this well	63, 67

P
Phisition doth well	36 until 50
Pirates undoes	102
Promotion spirituall	83
Pomeamber	49
Perfume	idem
Peace and unite	89
Prudence	35
Pestilence	37
Petty foggers	19
Purging the body	50

R

Rasis de peste	36
Ruf. contra pestem	41
Rogers writing	62
Rogers pleasant talke by the waye	60 &c.
Rewarde in Christ no merit in us	126
Resurrection of the dead	129

T

The iij. elementes	31
Trouble of mynde	26
The best remedy of the plague	44
To know the antrax	46
The tale of a Lion	63
The frutes of usury	11
The Lorde Crumwell	81
The discription of Ro. prela.	86
The Popes practise	87
The greatest crosse	117
The holy trinite	128
The holy churche	idem

W

Weomen have wormes in their tongues	102
Witchcrafte	104
What the soule is	33
We can cary nothing away	120
Wher it raineth double beer	101
Who shall shoe the mule	86
Who may not blede	41
Well fished	91

FINIS.

The manufacturer's authorised representative in the EU for product safety is Oxford University Press España S.A. of El Parque Empresarial San Fernando de Henares, Avenida de Castilla, 2 - 28830 Madrid (www.oup.es/en or product.safety@oup.com). OUP España S.A. also acts as importer into Spain of products made by the manufacturer.
Printed and bound by CPI Group (UK) Ltd, Croydon, CR0 4YY

31/03/2026

02081644-0001